Transformations in Queer, Trans, and Intersex Health and Aging

Breaking Boundaries: New Horizons in Gender & Sexualities

Series Editor: J. E. Sumerau, University of Tampa

Breaking Boundaries is meant to expand the horizons of mainstream and academic under-standings of sex, gender, and sexualities. While the last few decades have witnessed increased attention to some areas of sex, gender, and sexualities, mainstream and academic focus has been generally limited to focus on cissex males and females, cisgender women and men, monosexual gay/lesbian/straight, and monogamous individuals, groups, and experiences. Building on the groundwork laid by these traditions, Breaking Boundaries focuses on other arenas of sex, gender, and sexual identities, practices, relationships, experiences, and inequalities too often missing from existing mainstream and academic discussions of sex, gender, and sexualities.

Recent titles in the series:

Transformations in Queer, Trans, and Intersex Health and Aging

Alexandra C. H. Nowakowski,
J. E. Sumerau,
and Nik M. Lampe

LEXINGTON BOOKS
Lanham • Boulder • New York • London

Published by Lexington Books
An imprint of The Rowman & Littlefield Publishing Group, Inc.
4501 Forbes Boulevard, Suite 200, Lanham, Maryland 20706
www.rowman.com

6 Tinworth Street, London SE11 5AL, United Kingdom

British Library Cataloguing in Publication Information Available

Library of Congress Cataloging-in-Publication Data Available

ISBN: 9781793616340 (cloth)
ISBN: 9781793616364 (pbk)
Library of Congress Control Number: 2020942749

Contents

Introduction

It is 2018 in a large city in the Southeastern United States. A young, Hispanic, non-binary transgender person sits at a table in a bar with friends discussing the relief and joy they feel at finally interacting with medical providers who were able to respond to their health needs as a non-binary person in a positive way. They repeatedly thank the first author of this book, one of the friends at the table, who utilized their own medical expertise and experiences to recommend care plans as well as the clinic where they went to begin pursuing these plans. They recall, sometimes with a catch in their voice, how uncomfortable, frightening, and often painful other experiences with medical authorities have been before, and ask, as many have in various ways, what it might be like if medical professionals were better educated in terms of the empirical sex, gender, and sexual diversity of the world we live in and share.

A few days later, in another part of the city, the first author of this book reflects on the example shared above, and the ways they were able to use their knowledge, resources, and experience to help a friend gain adequate medical care. While at work that day, the first author of this book, as they often do, continues reviewing reports, responding on social media accounts, and making phone calls in their ongoing pursuit to help others obtain adequate care. At the same time, they continue working on their own research in this area as well as their work, professionally and personally, navigating life as an agender queer person with cystic fibrosis. In so doing, they begin to sketch out ideas for an upcoming presentation they will give to educate a group of medical students and other professionals on the varieties of sex, gender, and sexual identities, needs, and other health-related concerns.

At the same time the first author outlines their speech, the second author of this book stands in a college classroom in another city nearby where she teaches courses on sexualities, gender, health, and applied social science. It is early in the semester, and as usual, this means the second author stares out into a room of students who have generally never been taught much about the varieties of sex, gender, or sexualities in their lives to date. Many will not know what the words intersex or transgender mean, or much about safe sex, sexual minorities, healthy relationship practices, or many other aspects of sexual health. Some of them are becoming nurses, doctors, or other medical professionals, but even those may not have learned these basic aspects of sex, gender, and sexual experience that may become important in their careers and treatment of patients. As she does every semester, the second author of this book begins to outline the contours of sex, gender, and sexual variation as well as the ways such phenomena impact health and broader social life to a new group of students.

The next day, the third author of this book sits at a coffee shop back in the city where the friends sat in the bar only a few days before. There is a tape recorder running. They are sitting with a young, multiracial trans woman who agreed to be interviewed for a study exploring the healthcare experiences and needs of transgender and gender nonconforming youth. The third author of this book listens as their interviewee explains how frightening and difficult it is to go anywhere near any kind of medical office or setting due to negative treatment she has experienced in such places to date. She chokes up at times talking about how hard it is to just find medical practitioners who even understand basic aspects of transgender bodies, experiences, identities, or needs. She worries about the negative effects that may come from avoiding things like routine checkups because of the fear medical practitioners have created for her over time. The third author listens to each word, takes notes for their study, and even though they try not to, reflects upon their own negative experiences with medical practitioners lacking empathy, education, or both when faced with intersex, transgender, and/or queer patients.

Each of these examples reflect a common thread in contemporary discussions and debates at the intersection of sex, gender, and sexual health in the United States and more broadly (see, e.g., Johnson 2015; Pearce 2018; Sumerau and Mathers 2019). Put simply, researchers have increasingly begun to examine the ways that mainstream and historical forms of healthcare research, education, and practice are predicated upon assumptions about endosex (Davis 2015), cisgender (shuster 2018), and heterosexual (Schrock et al. 2014) norms and assumptions (see also Samuels 2014). Further, researchers have increasingly demonstrated negative effects mainstream medical models and norms have upon sex, gender, and sexual minorities. In fact, researchers have shown that medical efforts to limit sex, gender, and sexual possibilities into discrete, binary, and exclusive forms often justify and encourage the ongoing marginalization of sex, gender, and sexual minority groups (Costello 2019; Stryker 2008; Warner 1999).

As we have noted elsewhere (see, e.g., Lampe, Carter, and Sumerau 2019; Nowakowski and Sumerau 2019; Sumerau and Mathers 2019), such marginalization and erasure of sex, gender, and sexual variation in health mirrors and provides support for broader societal patterns of structure and behavior necessary for the maintenance of sex, gender, and sexual inequality (see also Schrock et al. 2014; Serano 2007; Warner 1999). When, for example, medical authorities erase or otherwise do away with bodies that do not conform to binary notions of male and female only, for example, they establish a foundational distinction in the treatment of human beings that can be used to justify differential treatment of such groups throughout society (Ridgeway 2011). Likewise, when medical authorities require conformity to a development model wherein all females become women and all males become men, they aid the erection and dissemination of a "cisgender reality" (Sumerau, Mathers, Cragun 2016) wherein any who deviate from said model are deemed unhealthy, abnormal, or otherwise problematic (Johnson 2015). Finally, when medical authorities define male-men and female-women as necessarily distinct beings who operate as halves or sides of a human whole, their efforts encourage and naturalize heterosexuality at the expense of other forms of sexual expression, desire, connection, and practice (Almeling 2011). In all such cases, medical erasure of sex, gender, and sexual variation creates and sustains societal patterns of sex, gender, and sexual inequalities.

As a result of these observations, emerging studies emphasizing the varieties or diversity of sex, gender, and sexual experiences, identities, practices, and bodies shed light upon many questions that remain unanswered in existing medical and other scientific literatures (see, e.g., Nowakowski and Sumerau 2019c; Nowakowski, Chan, Miller, Sumerau 2019; Taliaferro, Harder, Lampe, Carter, Rider, Eisenberg 2019 for recent reviews). Considering that the bulk of health and medical literature limits its focus to endosex assumptions, samples, or questions, what might we learn from more systematic consideration of intersex health over the life course (Davis 2015)? Similarly, since much of the research on lesbian, gay, bisexual, transgender, queer/questioning, intersex, and asexual (LGBTQIA) populations focuses explicitly on sexual health, what might we learn from the ways members of these populations navigate other aspects of health and medical practice (Johnson, Hill, Beach-Ferrara, Rogers, Bradford 2019)? Further, as much of the emerging work in transgender and intersex studies focuses on youth, what might we learn from the healthcare experiences of middle and later life transgender and intersex people (Sumerau and Mathers 2019)? While these are only a few of the questions emerging studies about variations in sex, gender, and sexual health may uncover (see also Santos, Pfeffer, Mann 2019), they reveal the importance of continued expansion and discussion of such variation in our hopes to understand and better provide healthcare for all populations regardless of where they fit within existing social norms.

Building on both our experiences as members of sex, gender, and/or sexual minority populations as well as our prior works in social and medical sciences, here we focus on some ways narrative and observational data culled from sex, gender, and/or sexual minority populations may provide insights into existing health disparities and potential avenues for future exploration and expansion of such fields. Throughout this book, we thus argue that, as has been the case every time previously hidden or erased populations have gained greater attention in society and the sciences (Samuels 2014), contemporary social and medical sciences face a pressing need to collect, analyze, and study experiences and narratives of sex, gender, and sexual health variation. Specifically, we utilize ourselves as case studies—in health as well as sex, gender, and sexual variation—in hopes of illuminating areas in need of systematic study for the potential betterment of health knowledge, practice, and education throughout society.

THE STUDY

In this book, we utilize ourselves as case studies for exploring some of the ways sex, gender, and sexual marginalization may impact health, healthcare access and experience, and understandings of the self over the life course. In developing this work, we drew upon studies noted above that reveal the need for greater illumination of the lived experiences of people who occupy marginalized sex, gender, and sexual social locations. For example, researchers have noted how emerging narrative studies of intersex populations reveal gaps and problems in existing medical procedures regarding birth, patient consent, and surgical practice (Roen 2008). In fact, such studies generally call for greater collection and analysis of the experiences of intersex people in relation to healthcare norms, expectations, and settings (Roen and Hegarty 2018). In this book, we follow such calls by providing specific narratives where sex, gender, and sexual experience intersect with the experience of health and medicine in complicated and nuanced ways less often captured in existing interdisciplinary socio-medical research (see also Nowakowski and Sumerau 2017b).

To this end, here we explicitly designed an exploratory study utilizing ourselves as case studies at the intersection of sex, gender, sexual, and health norms and assumptions. The first author, for example, engaged in an autoethnographic examination of their experiences as an agender, bisexual/queer, poly person navigating sex, relationships, and bodies in relation to their management of a chronic illness over time. The second author undertook an autoethnographic examination of her experiences navigating healthcare and management as a non-binary, bisexual, and poly trans woman who, for most of her life course to date, had very limited access to mainstream medical options for care. Finally, the third author undertook an autoethnographic study of their experiences managing bodily, emotional, and other forms of trauma in relation to their experiences as a non-binary, bisexual intersex person who did not learn about their intersex status until adulthood. In this way, here we provide three autoethnographic case studies that speak to both similar and varied experiences of intersections between sex, gender, sexual, and health experience over time and in relation to existing social norms.

As a result, this book relies heavily and builds upon interdisciplinary traditions of autoethnography as a method whereby in-depth consideration of a given case is used to create potential for further study (see, e.g., Adams 2011; Charmaz 2006; Crawley 2012; Lampe 2019a; Leavy 2015; Nowakowski 2017; Sumerau 2019 for discussion). Stated another way, we utilized autoethnographic efforts to outline missing pieces in existing interdisciplinary medical sciences, which could be further studied in qualitative, quantitative, historical, experiential, and/or arts-based methods over time (see also Rier 2000). As a method, autoethnography blends (1) ethnographic observation of a given subject, population, or social pattern in search of new insights to be gained from said observation (Geertz 1973) and (2) autobiographical analysis of the self as a case study in the experience of social life (Didion 2005). As such, autoethnography requires taking aspects of one's own life and examining such aspects in relation to existing artistic, scientific, and other forms of knowledge at a given time.

For the purposes of this book, we specifically utilized a tradition referred to as "collaborative autoethnography" (Chang et al. 2013). In simple terms, this tradition involves people doing autoethnographies of one or more subjects together (see Ellis and Rawicki 2013; Geist-Martin et al. 2010; Nowakowski and Sumerau 2019a for examples and discussion). Specifically, we each crafted separate autoethnographic analyses of our own intersections and experiences with health, sex, gender, and sexualities. Then, we utilized these individual analyses in collaborative revision and discussion to form this overall book as an exploration of potential future areas of research concerning intersections of sex, gender, sexuality, and health in contemporary U.S. society (see Methodological Appendix for further discussion). In so doing, we utilized both our individual experiences and insights and our collective reflection and analysis of the patterns within these individual accounts to form this book.

In this way, this book contains three separate, but interconnected case studies exploring potential ways sex, gender, sexuality, and health may play out in the lived experiences of people who occupy sex, gender, and/or sexual minority locations. As such, our work here provides an exploration of potential pathways for future studies seeking to better understand or potentially change existing sex, gender, and sexual norms within health and medicine as well as observations that may guide the formation of interview and survey instruments for future study of sex, gender, and sexual minorities navigating healthcare. In fact, we return to these types of questions in each chapter and complete the work by drawing out implications from the combination of our experiences for future interdisciplinary studies of health and healthcare experience over the life course and in relation to multiple social locations.

From this starting point, our study here thus explores the ways sex, gender, and sexual variation may become relevant in the experience of health, healthcare, and medical interactions over the life course. While more and more surveys demonstrate significant disparities in healthcare outcomes and experiences in relation to sex, gender, and sexualities (Calasanti and Slevin 2001; Harder and Sumerau 2019; Nowakowski and Sumerau 2015), here we dig into the nuances and complexities of how people may experience such patterns. Likewise, as increasing qualitative studies point to barriers and concerns about healthcare access for sex, gender, and sexual minorities (Davis 2015; Johnson and Rogers 2019; shuster 2017; Sumerau and Mathers 2019), here we explore the effects of such difficulties on the ways people experience their health, sex, gender, and sexuality over time. Throughout this book, we argue that examining the complexities and nuances of sex, gender, sexual, and health experiences necessitates an ongoing expansion and exploration of our existing socio-medical theoretical and methodological traditions, subject areas, and overall foci to better include the varieties of sex, gender, and sexuality.

Sex, Gender, and Sexual Health

Before turning to our analyses in the autoethnographic chapters of this book, it is important to examine existing work on intersections between sex, gender, sexuality, and health. Although entire books are written on each of these four topics and some of the ways they impact one another in varied settings, here we focus on important patterns necessary for both considering the autoethnographic analyses presented here, and the possibilities for future research expanding upon existing knowledge. To this end, we focus this section on the ways sex, gender, and sexualities have been shown to impact health, healthcare, medicine, and other related phenomena in a wide variety of settings, contexts, and ways over time.

To this end, we begin with the social construction of endosex as the only normal formation of sex status, identity, and characteristic by medical authorities over time (see Costello 2019; Davis 2015; Roen 2008; Topp 2019 for reviews). Stated simply, medical authorities in the United States and many other countries established discrete, mutually exclusive sex categories that were labeled male and female (Samuels 2014). Then, the same authorities argued that all humans should be placed into one or the other of these categories at birth even though biological characteristics referred to as sex have always been more varied and expansive than any two categories (Karzakis 2008). In so doing, medical and other social authorities created what we call "sex" as a location within male or female categories based on the appearance of genitals.

Scholars refer to those people who "fit neatly" into these male/female exclusive categorizations as endosex. Endosex people are assigned male or female, and often think very little about this assignment—or the possibility that it was incorrect in any biologically empirical way—throughout their lives unless something unexpected forces them to consider it. Although people often talk about chromosomes, hormones, and other biological factors in media, religion, sciences, and other arenas, these factors are rarely involved in the assignment of people to endosex categories at birth (Davis 2015). Rather, such assignment is typically carried out based on appearance and models for what is considered "normal" genital appearance. In this way, medical authorities create sex each time they assign a baby to a given category.

As suggested above, many unexpected events may occur over time in one's life to demonstrate the socially constructed nature of sex, but for the purposes of this book, here we focus on categorization itself. Just as people are categorized as endosex if they fit into socially agreed upon notions of male and female appearance at birth, others are categorized as intersex if they do not fit into these notions (Costello 2019). Although there are a wide variety of ways one may be deemed intersex or may claim intersex as an identity, medical authorities typically define or assign babies as such based on the observation of some "abnormal" element of genital or other appearance. In such cases, intersex children are often subjected to unnecessary surgeries to force them into the appearance of an endosex body (Davis 2015). These surgeries often also cause negative effects in terms of reproductive, sexual, and other capabilities for the children as they age, but have thus far been shown to have no medical or health benefits for the children.

The implications from the paragraphs above play out in significant ways when it comes to both health and other experiences of social life. Researchers have repeatedly found, for example, that one's assignment as male or female often serves as a fundamental or overwhelming cause of much of one's biological and social experience as well as a primary axis wherein some receive better treatment than others (see, e.g., Harder and Sumerau 2019; Nowakowski, Graves, and Sumerau 2016; Read and Gorman 2010 for recent reviews). We would call this "within endosex health disparities" wherein endosex female and endosex male people often experience disparate health outcomes. At the same time, researchers increasingly demonstrate that intersex people experience significant health disparities in comparison to endosex people (see, e.g., Costello 2019; Davis 2015; Roen 2008). These we might refer to as "health disparities between endosex and intersex people" or simply "sex disparities in health" wherein intersex or endosex assignment itself creates negative mental and/or physical health outcomes for people over time. However we name such patterns, research demonstrates that sex, as a socially constructed axis of meaning, creates and reproduces variations in the health experiences and outcomes of people (Almeling 2011).

Of course, since sex assignment is typically utilized by medical authorities and the public to assign children to a given gender identity (i.e., it's a boy!) (West and Zimmerman 1987), these inequalities only become more complicated and nuanced when we turn to gender. Stated simply, most medical professionals and parents will build on the sex assignment of a child (i.e., that is an endosex male) to further assign the child with a gender identity (i.e., endosex males are boys and should become men over time) (Sumerau 2020). This process may be referred to as the creation of a cisgender identity, or the expectation that one will conform to a given gender identity based upon their assignment to a given sex category (Sumerau and Mathers 2019). In fact, much health research follows this same cisgender identity creation process by using sex (i.e., respondent is male or female on a survey) as a proxy for gender (i.e., male respondent is measured as man) in their analyses (see, e.g., Nowakowski et al. 2016; Sumerau et al. 2017; Westbrook and Saperstein 2015). As West and Zimmerman (1987) note, this is because the assumption of a required path between sex assignment as conforming to a specific gender identity is embedded throughout every aspect of contemporary society (see also Goffman 1977).

As a result, we not surprisingly find similar health disparities between people who identify or are assigned female as we do among people who identify as or are assigned as women in most research studies (see Calasanti and Slevin 2001 for review). Countless studies find that assigned-female at birth people who identify as women (i.e., cisgender women) and cisgender men (i.e., people assigned male who identify as men) differ significantly in many areas of mental, physical, chronic, and acute health outcomes throughout the life course (see, e.g., Bird 1999; Harder and Sumerau 2019; Hill and Needham 2013 for reviews). Further, researchers have noted that the ways cisgender women and cisgender men approach health often follow societal assumptions about what it means to be a man or woman and how such men or women should behave in society (see Courtenay 2000; Cragun and Sumerau 2017; Needham and Hill 2010). Overall, researchers consistently find that gender itself, within cisgender populations, operates as a primary cause of specific health outcomes. We might refer to these patterns as "within cisgender health disparities," but current health research typically refers to them only as "gender inequalities" because cisgender privilege remains normal and assumed even in scientific studies and language norms (Serano 2007).

At the same time, however, more recent scholarship expands to "gender inequalities" overall, and in so doing, demonstrates significant variation in health outcomes, experiences, and even access between cisgender populations, on the one hand, and transgender, gender non-conforming, and non-binary (i.e., whether or not they identify as transgender or gender non-conforming as well) populations on the other hand (see, e.g., Johnson and Rogers 2019; Miller and Grollman 2015; Sumerau and Mathers 2019). Transgender and other gender variant (i.e., non-cisgender identified) people report, for example, difficulties accessing medical care, significant negative physical and mental effects due to individual and structural patterns of transphobia in society, and inadequate information and education on the part of medical "professionals" in terms of transgender and other non-cisgender bodies, healthcare needs, medical protocols, and health options (see also Johnson and Rogers 2019). Researchers thus document societal wide disparities between cisgender and transgender populations. Such studies also find "within cisgender" disparities in health outcomes, experiences, and expectations, but further add recognition of inequalities between cisgender and gender variant populations, and "within gender variant" disparities (i.e., differences in health between transgender and otherwise gender variant populations). In so doing, these studies begin to study "gender inequalities" in health rather than disparities within only one specific gender population.

At the same time, however, health and medical disparities also arise due to the cisgender assumptions of medical norms at present. As noted above, most doctors and parents build on the assignment of sex (i.e., it's an endosex male) to require children to conform to a specific gender identity (i.e., it's a boy) (see Sumerau 2020 for discussion). Transgender, gender non-conforming, and non-binary people, however, all reject this cisgender identity pathway rather than conforming to it (Johnson 2015). Although such people may diverge from this pathway at any time in the life course or in a wide variety of ways, the divergence leaves them outside the cisgender assumptions of society (West and Zimmerman 1987) and modern medicine (Samuels 2014) even as they must navigate these assumptions in their own lives (Ashley 2019a; 2019b; Johnson 2015; Sumerau and Mathers 2019). This means gender variant people automatically fall outside the normal confines of what doctors and parents define as a healthy pathway of development (Johnson 2015). Despite the many similarities and differences that exist within and between varied transgender, gender non-conforming, non-binary, or otherwise gender variant populations, people in each group face this outsider status in relation to normative medical protocols, and thus members of these groups become more likely to experience negative health outcomes through the initial creation of sex and gender by medical authorities.

Although the paragraphs above already reveal a complex interplay between sex, gender, and health, sexuality poses yet another nuanced, complex arena necessary for understanding the experiences of people in relation to medical norms (Foucault 1978; Halkitis 2013; Orne and Gall 2019). One reason for this is that non-heterosexual sexualities (Schrock et al. 2014), non-endosex sexes (Davis 2015), and non-cisgender genders (Styrker 2008) have each been defined as diseased or otherwise unhealthy by medical authorities at different times in history (see also Warner 1999). This is also because sexual health and education programs have consistently been the source of political conflicts, debates, and concerns throughout the past century (see, e.g., Fields 2008; Elliott 2012; Heath 2012). In fact, there are very few aspects of contemporary medical and otherwise health-related practice that do not, in some way, rely upon and develop in response to prior, shifting, and existing sexual norms and assumptions (Almeling 2011).

One way this becomes especially salient in the health-related experiences, outcomes, and other aspects of people's lives involves the construction and promotion of heterosexuality as normal, natural, and healthy by medical authorities throughout, at least, the past century (see Schrock et al. 2014 for review). To revisit our discussions above, note that (1) people are sorted into sex categories created and enforced by medical authorities and based on genitals; and (2) people are then required or expected to conform to gender identities based on these initial sex and genital categorizations. In this way, medical authorities have already defined what will count as so called normal, natural, healthy heterosexuality for any given baby—it will involve attraction and desire for other humans who were assigned differently in terms of sex and then expected to conform to a different gender identity than the baby in question.

Since heterosexuality, like homosexuality (i.e., monosexual identities, see Barringer et al. 2017), is predicated upon genital and/or sex and gender sameness/difference, medical authorities' assignment of babies to one or another sex and gender category creates what "heterosexuality" will mean for that specific baby. This is because the twin actions of sex and gender assignment will define the socially sanctioned object of desire that baby will be expected to develop. Put simply, without the initial segregation of babies into sex and gender categories, monosexuality (i.e., sexual desire predicated upon one type of sex or gender only) cannot exist, and therefore, heterosexuality as social norm and requirement has no foundation for its existence (Warner 1999). This observation may not matter to one who feels comfortable in their sex, gender, and sexuality (i.e., comfortable with their endosex, cisgender, mono-heterosexual assignment), but it creates considerable inequality and difficulty for anyone who does not fit any or all of these assumptions (see Schrock et al. 2014 for examples throughout society).

Not surprisingly, researchers have picked up on these observations in increasingly common studies of sexual disparities in health. Specifically, such studies find that heterosexual, cisgender women typically experience significant health inequalities in comparison to heterosexual cisgender men, that lesbian and gay people (i.e., monosexual minorities) regardless of sex and gender identities often face significant health disparities in relation to heterosexual people, that bisexual/pansexual/queer/fluid people (i.e., non-monosexual people) face significant disparities in relation to some lesbian/gay monosexual people and to monosexual heterosexual people in particular, and that asexual people (i.e., non-monosexual and non-sexual identified people) often experience significant disparities in relation to all of these other populations (see, for review, Simula, Miller, and Sumerau 2019; Sumerau and Mathers 2019). In each case, people who deviate in one or more ways from the sex, gender, sexual pathway promoted and created as normal by medical authorities typically face negative consequences as a result.

In fact, we can see the widespread impact of monosexual and heterosexual assumptions embedded into existing healthcare and other medical systems in many different areas of research. In terms of reproductive healthcare, for example, researchers demonstrate how assumptions about heterosexuality permeate even the terminology utilized by medical professionals and patients (Almeling 2011). Likewise, studies show significant increases in negative health outcomes including but not limited to substance abuse, anxiety, stress, suicidal ideation, coronary problems, access to adequate care, and care for later life among sex, gender, and sexual minority communities throughout the United States (see Nowakowski et al. 2019 for review). Similarly, researchers have shown how assumptions about endosex, cisgender, heterosexuality in medical education leave many medical practitioners lacking in their abilities to handle routine interactions with patients who do not fit these assumptions in terms of identities, bodies, or both (see, for reviews, Davis 2015; Johnson 2015; Sumerau and Mathers 2019). In all such cases, sexual variations combine with sex and gender variations to create a scenario where those who fit social norms receive better healthcare and generally have better health outcomes than those who do not fit such norms.

In this book, we thus draw on each of these ongoing lines of research to examine specific ways sex, gender, and sexualities intersect in the health-related experiences of people over the life course. Specifically, we utilize ourselves as case studies often less common in existing research to draw out potential future directions and areas of study for each of these topic areas. To this end, we seek to build on the ongoing works of scholars throughout the arts and sciences as we, each in our own ways, seek to transform existing medical and social norms from systems predicated upon fitting a specific, narrow model into systems where all people may find care for the needs, identities, and experiences of their lives regardless of social location. With this in mind, we provide an overview of the discussions to come in the following section.

Organization of the Book

With the aforementioned considerations in mind, we turn to the first autoethnographic analysis in chapter 1. Specifically, the first author outlines how sex, gender, and sexual experiences intersect with health and well-being as an agender, bisexual, poly person managing a chronic health condition and an active sexual and romantic life. In so doing, the first author outlines some ways that sexual norms shift in relation to the management of a chronic health condition as well as the ways sex and gender identities may impact such management. Further, they posit aspects of health, sex, gender, sexual identity, and sexual practice that may be more or less relevant in relation to different experiences of what it means to be healthy, sexual, and romantic as a result of different bodily forms and expectations. In so doing, the first author draws attention to the nexus of health status and sex/gender/sexual/ health practice over time.

In chapter 2, we move into other variations of sex, gender, and sexuality as the second author encourages the acceptance and understanding of complexity in notions of health and aging. Specifically, she outlines some ways her experiences as a non-binary, bisexual, and poly trans woman who grew up in the working and lower classes facilitated specific strategies for navigating health in relation to class disadvantage, trauma, and gender complexity. Further, she outlines the ways resources, or lack thereof, complicate such relationships over time, and some ways that assumptions about sex, gender, sexual, and health meanings and norms take different forms in relation to race, class, and other social locations. In so doing, she outlines potential benefits from embracing the complexity of lived experience in our attempts to understand health and design systems of healthcare.

Turning to our third autoethnographic analyses in chapter 3, the third author examines how medical assumptions, knowledges, and norms shift in relation to unexpected changes over the life course. Specifically, the third author discusses how their experiences as a non-binary, bisexual, intersex person influenced their varying notions of bodies, health-related habits, trauma experience and recovery, and interactions with medicine over time. Moreover, they discuss some ways learning about intersex status in adulthood may impact how one views experiences of sex, gender, sexual, and health intersections earlier in life. In so doing, the third author draws attention to nuances of intersex sex, gender, and sexual experience as well as the importance of studying how intersex people experience health and aging over time.

After presenting these three autoethnographic examinations of intersections between sex, gender, sexualities, and health, we draw out implications from the combination of these insights in the final chapter of the book. Specifically, we ask what aspects of our similar and different experiences navigating sex, gender, sexualities, and health might advance existing health research, studies of intersex health and aging, transgender and queer focused research, and examinations of how people age with chronic conditions and in relation to sexual desires. We further explore other potential avenues wherein our individual and collective experiences suggest there may still be much to learn about the nuances and complexities of sex, gender, and sexual experience in relation to health and other social systems. In closing, we address each of these issues in relation to potential future studies and theoretical implications for our understanding of the social and medical construction of health, sex, gender, and sexualities over time.

Chapter One

You're Rubber, I'm Glue

*Navigating Changing Meanings of
Safe Sex with Cystic Fibrosis*

I have cystic fibrosis (CF). I also frequently have sex. Whether or not this is surprising depends on your point of view. Once upon a time, my being thirty-five-years old and thriving reasonably well with CF would have been shocking. Today, this is hardly out of the ordinary. Health and longevity for people with CF, a genetic disease that causes problems with a protein that helps to move substances across cell membranes, has changed tremendously during my lifetime (Nowakowski 2018a). Our median life expectancy has risen to forty-seven years for patients based in the United States and continues to climb with each passing year. CF remains a complex and challenging chronic disease to manage, as it basically turns the body's mucus into rubber cement. But as more patients live longer and healthier lives, we increasingly enjoy a wide variety of "normal" adult experiences. For many of us, this includes sexual relationships of various types and durations.

People often think of CF as a lung disease, but it actually impacts the entire body. The same issues with sticky, viscous mucus that harm our lungs also affect other mucous membranes. These include the intestines, the bladder, the kidneys, and—you guessed it—the genitals (Nowakowski 2018a). The outer membranes of our genital regions thus do not work quite the same way they would if we did not have CF. Instead of making thin fluid to lubricate the membranes, our genitals produce that same tacky substance reminiscent of rubber cement. Predictably, this does not facilitate comfortable or safe sex. So, because we are "glue" in the sense that our bodies' natural lubrication functions as more of an adhesive, we often benefit from resources that help us keep the membranes slick and damp. Likewise, we also tend to benefit from prophylaxis for infection (Nowakowski 2018b). This can include wiping with antibacterial towelettes before and after sexual activity and using condoms for vaginal or anal penetration—the "rubber" part of this analogy. To put things bluntly, if I want to have vaginal intercourse for any substantial amount of time, I need to use lots of lube and have my partner use a condom.

With a few notable exceptions, little literature currently exists on sexuality among people with CF specifically. This may owe in part to historically poor survival among affected individuals. Without many people aging into adulthood with CF or sharing openly about that experience in generations past, the idea that people with this disease could have lengthy and active sexual lives took time to proliferate in public knowledge, let alone academic research. However, a diverse and nuanced literature absolutely exists on the broader topic of chronic illness and sexuality. This body of work intersects with scholarship on related issues such as sexuality and identity as well as meaning-making in sexual relationships. I draw heavily on these literatures in exploring transformations in my own awareness of my sexuality and what it means for me to practice "safe sex" as a person with CF.

My experiences with CF, both more broadly and then specifically as they relate to my sexual biography, also do not exist in a vacuum. These experiences are situated firmly in and impacted substantially by my contexts as a person of queer (bi and pan sexual) sexuality and nonbinary gender identity. For me, being queer means having attractions to people of a variety of sex and gender identities and presentations. There has also been some variation in the sexes of my partners, though at least thus far everyone I have been intimate with has had a penis during at least part of the time I was with them. As I have learned more about the nuances of sexuality in the course of my own work and lived experience, I have realized that I am best described as bisexual or pansexual in practice and begun describing myself this way while remaining attentive to shared experiences within the broader queer community. I have also become more open in narrating my precise location within the nonbinary landscape: I am agender. This aspect of my identity also automatically introduces an element of queerness into all of my relationships, regardless of the gender or sex identity of a particular partner. For me, being agender means not having an intrinsic sense of myself as a gendered being while simultaneously realizing that others often see me in gendered ways. So, my intersecting identities as someone of female sex, nonexistent gender, and queer sexuality absolutely shape my experiences of intimacy with CF.

My physical health experiences likewise interact dynamically with my experiences as a partner in both an open marriage with a nonbinary trans woman (i.e., the second author of this book) and a nonmarital relationship with a cisgender man. Yet as with other literatures on health and related experiences, awareness of and attention to the nuances of wellness and intimacy for populations outside the cisgender and heterosexual social norms has developed slowly. This poses problems not only from a diversity and inclusion perspective, but also from a knowledge and implementation one. People of non-cis and non-hetero biographies often have particular experiences in our sexual lives that intertwine with the multiple marginalization we face in other areas. Moreover, we also experience elevated risk for sexual abuse and other forms of intimate partner violence, and for catastrophic harm from such abusive situations. So, I have increasingly centered concepts of non-hetero sexuality and non-cis gender experience in my own work on living and aging with chronic disease, and how my own journey with CF can inform broader inquiry on such questions.

My prior work in this area has engaged my personal biography with CF in several intersecting ways. In "Hope Is a Four Letter Word," I outlined the dualistic nature of optimism in life course journeys with chronic disease through the lens of taking a new medication to combat dryness in my mucous membranes (Nowakowski 2016a). In "You Poor Thing," I explored the infantilization and desexualization of people with visible chronic conditions (Nowakowski 2016b; see also Gill 2015). In "Neverland," I examined the often quixotic experience of aging with CF and my own unique perspectives on that journey as someone who remains relatively young overall (Nowakowski 2019a). In "The Salt without the Girl," I challenged the stereotyping of both people with CF and people with nonbinary gender identity, and how those experiences intersect uniquely in the context of queer sexuality (Nowakowski 2019b). And in "Reframing Health and Illness," I analyzed the dynamic nature of understanding one's own journey with chronic disease and medical diagnosis (Nowakowski and Sumerau 2019a). I collaborated on the "Reframing Health and Illness" manuscript with my spouse, an expert ethnographer and also the second author of this book (see also Nowakowski and Sumerau 2017a). This collaborative inquiry process facilitated critical examination of our relationships to one another, including in relation to our individual and collective sexualities.

In this book chapter, I build on this prior body of work by synthesizing scholarship on chronic disease, sexual activity, and intersectional marginalization in the context of life course illness transformations. As in previous pieces like "The Salt without the Girl" (Nowakowski 2019b), I use anecdotes from my own lived experience to offer autoethnographic guidance for critical review of relevant literature (see Methodological Appendix for discussion of Autoethnography). I then reflect on enduring gaps in published research and highlight opportunities for further scholarship.

EXAMINING STANDPOINT

As a person with CF living in the United States, I am part of a small population—about thirty thousand people nationwide. This compares to the total
national population size of around 350 million people. Being part of such a
small and insular community absolutely makes me see the world differently.
And as many others with CF will tell you, our patient population truly is a
community. We share many characteristics and are also often much more
diverse than people realize. For example, although we are a small population,
we are also a microcosm of humanity as a whole. People of any racial
identity, ethnic affiliation, cultural background, or geographic origin can
have CF. All you need to have the disease is some combination of problems
with the production, transport, and/or functioning of your CFTR proteins as
described above. Because of this, people with CF are a diverse community in
ways that go well beyond race, ethnicity, culture, and origin. The fact that
our population includes people of different sexes, genders, and sexualities
has been particularly relevant for my own experience.

Within that small community of people diagnosed with CF in the United
States, I occupy several other minority locations by virtue of being openly
queer, agender, and polyamorous. I have grown accustomed in various areas
of my life to often being the first person in a group to disclose one or more of
these identities. My experiences within the CF community have thus far
proven to be no exception. Yet through social media I have been fortunate to
meet and bond with others who share some or all of these characteristics.
These experiences have made me feel much less isolated in my own journey
with the disease, and more hopeful about my future as I continue to age.

I am also in some ways an island because of the specific genetic characteristics associated with my particular case of CF. Presently there are over
2,300 known gene variants associated with at least one documented clinical
case of the disease. However, about 80 percent of the global CF population
has one copy of a common mutation: a deletion at location 508F on the
CFTR gene. When I finally had my CFTR genes sequenced at age 33, my
care team found one copy of c.1584+36A<G, a substitution on one of the two
genes. I also do not have any copies of the 508F deletion. This places me in
two unique populations within the CF community: individuals with rare mutations and phenotypically classic patients with only one CFTR mutation.
Cases like mine have helped scientists and clinicians alike to learn about the
origins of CF and how it can best be managed in people with different
individual disease characteristics, including genetic mutations. My unique
genetics may also help to explain why I survived as long as I did without
receiving comprehensive, guideline-based CF care for most of my life.

More than fifteen thousand members of the national CF patient population are presently over eighteen years of age—a milestone we only reached

in 2017. This means that getting older with CF continues to make people outliers within an already small community. In 2019, only perhaps 10 percent of people with CF in the United States are over the age of 40. Barring any major setbacks with my care—always a hypothetical statement, even if a hopeful one—I will celebrate my fortieth birthday at the end of 2023. At 35, I have already outlived many of my generational peers with the disease. This has increasingly made me a voice, in both my professional practice and the general community, for the clinical relevance of attention to aging with CF.

Given the persistence of CF in compressing the lifespans of many people who live with it, it should come as little surprise that historically our family members have played key roles in amplifying our stories. We are thankfully transitioning within the U.S. health system from viewing CF as a pediatric disease to a chronic progressive one that may involve survival to very old ages—just as a more capricious and complex journey than it otherwise would. But historically, our family members often spoke for us because as children we could not legally speak for ourselves in medical decision-making scenarios. In the present day, we often still rely on our family members to advocate for us even as we raise our own voices in the care planning and implementation process. The same occurs in a variety of other activities such as lobbying that extend far beyond the boundaries of direct clinical care. As more of us survive farther into adulthood, our teams of advocates often include intimate partners.

I myself have been married twice—once to someone who was not an active participant in my healthcare and presently to someone who very much is. I receive assistance with several specific types of care activities from my spouse, including airway clearance and medication management. I also provide support to her in kind as she deals with a number of other chronic health challenges (see chapter 3 for more information). And my spouse provides an enormous depth and breadth of emotional and social support—more than I could possibly enumerate or quantify. This reciprocal process of caregiving presents itself as much in the physically intimate aspects of our relationship as it does in all others, with each of us consistently monitoring the other person's experience and well-being (see Nowakowski and Sumerau 2017a). With my CF, this proves especially important in particular ways related to the stickiness of my mucus, the ease with which the underlying membranes become infected, and the scar tissue created by past infections. It also matters in relation to prior injuries that resulted from other people's devaluation of my own health.

Caregiving for one another with respect to sexual wellness comes easily for me and my spouse in part because both of us have survived sexual abuse. Our experiences of post-traumatic stress from sexual violation stem from very different origins, but have similar consequences and impacts on our shared dynamic as partners. Over almost ten years together, my spouse and I have built a comprehensive culture of affirmative consent that extends well beyond our explicitly sexual activities. We value the outstanding support we receive from one another on every front, including but certainly not limited to sexuality. Our shared history of abuse makes us all the more conscious of and grateful for what we share together. I have met many other people in the CF community with similar personal histories of experiencing abuse. This includes stories about partners willfully disregarding safety precautions necessary to keep the person with CF healthy as "unromantic," and messaging about people with CF being "lucky" to garner sexual interest from anyone because we are sick. My own history with abuse exposed me to both of these types of experiences, as well as others. I have also found these experiences to be particularly common among relatively older members of the adult CF community. This may owe somewhat to improved understanding of what constitutes safe sex for people with CF—a journey I and others are still on. It may also stem partly from increased general social awareness of sexual abuse, as evidenced by the #MeToo movement (see O'Neil et al. 2018 for discussion of #MeToo in relation to health) and other key developments in public discourse on consent.

As suggested previously, I am also often sexually active in other relationships outside of my marriage. My spouse and I have always practiced openness, although whether or not either of us had other partners at a given time has varied across the nearly decade-long span of our partnership. Both in itself and as it relates to my CF, our shared practice of nonmonogamy—what we referred to as "relational fluidity" in a prior manuscript (Sumerau and Nowakowski 2019)—introduces additional parameters for safe sexual contact. For example, concern about cross-infection means that anyone who wishes to become involved sexually with either one of us must agree not to pursue physical intimacy with other CF patients. The presence of different partners also introduces different individual sexual dynamics that may require different safety precautions within each relationship. For example, the "rubber" bit implicated in the title of this chapter becomes vastly more important in partnerships where I have more vaginal intercourse.

While enjoying physical intimacy within my marriage itself, I also contend with the different forms of marginalization my spouse and I have experienced that intersect with the additional constraints imposed by my CF. Which aspects of our individual and shared experiences prove most salient within a particular activity or context can vary greatly. My CF is thus not always the primary factor shaping our sexual dynamic, though it always enters into the equation somehow. On a broader level, this variability has frequently spurred both of us to reflect on the fact that who serves as the caregiver and who serves as the care recipient in these contexts is always relative, and highly dynamic as well. We have reflected on this in a general sense with respect to health challenges and caregiving, and in a specific one with respect to partners' experiences of aging together with chronic disease, in our collaborative scholarship.

Exploration of evolving sexuality in people living and aging with CF within the context of their intimate partnerships brings reciprocal caregiving "out of the shadow" in ways that offer unique value for clinical and community health management (Nowakowski and Sumerau 2017a).

I thus devote the remainder of this chapter to exploring these concepts in the specific context of my experiences of being sexual while managing CF. In the process, I review and synthesize relevant contributions from prior research on chronic disease and sexuality. I also compare and contrast my own experiences with those of others I have met in my own journey through aging with CF. This includes both individuals living with CF themselves and those managing other chronic conditions. I organize these reflections by several major themes suggested in this introductory exploration of standpoint: dichotomies between sickness and sexiness; perceptions of the body being disgusting; constant threats of infection; painful experiences and the toughness they instill; and sex as a contextually situated experience.

TO BE SICK OR TO BE SEXY

Public discourse on chronic disease often suggests a dichotomy between sickness and sexiness. This dichotomy becomes particularly apparent in dialogue about older people. Aging exposes people to a certain amount of social desexualization even in scenarios of relatively good general health. In situations where aging involves either the onset of a new illness or the progression of an existing one, desexualization intensifies. Scholars of long-term care have written extensively about this issue. Prior literature describes phenomena like the forced separation of long-term intimate partners in skilled nursing facilities, and the perception that people with mild cognitive impairment have no capacity for sexual consent.

Even in cases of aging with chronic illness managed in outpatient settings, a general narrative of growing older as losing sexuality persists. Contrasting narratives presented about HIV/AIDS in populations of different ages offer a vivid example. Nursing home staff have often reacted with surprise to the discovery of sexually acquired HIV infections among their patients. Yet when children in the late twentieth century received transfusions of HIV-infected blood, peer groups and media narratives alike quickly suggested sexual activity as the cause of their declining health. And in middle age populations living with HIV/AIDS, often the concept that people with this group of health conditions could be sexy pervaded public consciousness via images of people like basketball star Magic Johnson who did not "look sick" in any outward way. The reification of narratives surrounding people's ability to remain sexy while living with HIV/AIDS continued to center on normative constructions of the sexual body, and still does.

Aging with chronic illness thus introduces expectations of performing illness as a removal of self from sexual spheres and roles. In the case of CF specifically, the example of HIV/AIDS offers particularly apt insight. Although HIV and AIDS are infectious diseases rather than genetic ones, both have historically been considered both progressive conditions and terminal ones. In the present, innovations in treatment have offered many people living with both conditions the chance to slow down the progression of their disease tremendously. Likewise, numerous people with both HIV and CF are now living long lives—especially in cases where they can consistently access quality healthcare. And as more people impacted by either CF or HIV in childhood age into sexual maturity, our experiences demand a reckoning with notions of lifelong chronic illness as a barrier to sexuality.

Aging into sexual maturity with CF also implies questions of adaptive sexuality and the ability of people with disabling conditions to be sexy. The general disability literature offers abundant examples of how abled people often desexualize their peers, especially those with visible physical impairment (Gill 2015). Literature on specific degenerative conditions that involve changes in physical functioning, such as multiple sclerosis and Parkinson's disease, offer particularly sharp insights into perceptions of sexuality in aging with progressive physical disease. This discourse often appears in popular media as well. In *Love and Other Drugs*, protagonist Maggie has early-onset Parkinson's disease. She feels doubtful and suspicious of her partner's interest in being with her, asking if he feels good about himself because he "pity fucked the sick girl" and suggesting that a sexual relationship with her might feel more like penitence than privilege.

Yet *Love and Other Drugs* also offers examples of the complex interplay between different types of body privilege. Although Maggie has physical functioning challenges, she is also young, thin, white, presented-as-straight, and played by a performer (Anne Hathaway) whom many consider to be very attractive. Her story contrasts sharply with that of Dotty in *Cloudburst*, whose longtime same-sex partner must fight tirelessly to demonstrate that she remains a social and sexual being whose humanity would be erased by institutionalization. Dotty (played by Brenda Fricker) is much older than Maggie, with none of the physical trappings generally deemed "sexy" in the contemporary United States. The film thus encourages audiences to challenge notions of older adults as automatically nonsexual, vibrantly centers the sexual appeal and energy of people with diverse bodies aging into later life, and refutes the idea that people with chronic conditions cannot be desirable.

Several members of the CF community have played instrumental roles in turning conventional thinking about sickness and sexuality inside out. Perhaps the most prominent example is Bob Flanagan, the performance artist who used BDSM practice to explore social meanings of illness and death. Flanagan was profiled in the documentary *Sick: The Life and Death of Bob Flanagan, Supermasochist* and also featured in several music videos for Nine Inch Nails. These media explore Flanagan's use of ruthless corporeal play to master an unruly body. In Flanagan's visual art, his frail appearance becomes part and parcel of his sexual intrigue. This occurs partly via the contrast between his slight body and his ability to perform incredible feats of masochism, such as enduring full days in total bondage and nailing his foreskin to a wooden board. His narration of his physical exploration of sexuality invokes many of the same principles I incorporated in "You Poor Thing"—especially the idea of the element of surprise as a core component of autonomous sexuality in living with visible chronic disease (Nowakowski 2016b).

Unsurprisingly, Flanagan's hypersexual approach to aging with CF may read differently than the same behavior would in someone with a different variety of progressive disease—or just someone with CF who remains pancreatic sufficient and thus lacks the slender physical appearance often associated with the condition. Although Flanagan appears frail in much of his visual work, he still retains thin privilege as well as intersecting social advantages of whiteness and educational attainment. Body diversity exists in the CF community just as it does in other communities of people aging with progressive disease. But likewise, established norms of attractiveness and desirability related to body size and shape appear just as surely in our community as they do in the general population.

Ian Pettigrew's photo series *Salty Girls*—a collection of photographs of women, females, and femmes living with CF—showcases both the general tendency of patients to be thinner and some specific examples of patients who are much heavier. The fact that Pettigrew has CF himself adds an additional layer of nuance. Indeed, *Salty Girls* has become even more instructive on the interplay between CF, aging, and sexiness in recent years as Pettigrew has publicly documented his own journey with bodybuilding. He sometimes posts photos of his physical progress on his blog and reflects openly about how he feels more attractive and desirable now. I explored some of these same dynamics in "The Salt without the Girl" through the lens of an almost weaponized disinterest in adhering to established norms of sexiness as mutually exclusive with frailty (Nowakowski 2019b). I suppose it comes as no surprise that my favorite *Salty Girls* models are the ones proudly showing their bones with defiant expressions on their faces.

Written and visual narratives of aging with CF neatly capture general notions of the unruly and intractable body that pervade broader discourse on chronic illness, sexual behavior, and the life course. The desire to master the body and make it behave—whether in "normal" ways or superhuman ones—appears prominently in diverse descriptions of living and aging with CF in multiple forms of media. Dialogue about believing in oneself as a sexual being often intertwines with this discourse, sometimes with humor and sometimes with sorrow. I have experienced both in ample quantities on my own journey through the life course. In "You Poor Thing" I described an encounter where a person stopped attempting to flirt with me the moment they realized I was sick (Nowakowski 2016b). Yet I also see a different view of my own sexuality every day in my marriage. My spouse has repeatedly and explicitly stated that nothing my body does as a result of my CF could ever make it less sexy in her eyes. As she has spent many hours cleaning up various products of the same, including the impressive amount of vomit I managed to get all over our bathroom after one of my surgeries, I feel inclined to believe her. These discussions have also given me deep awareness of how the concept of "grossness" plays into notions of sexuality among people aging with CF and other chronic diseases.

ON BEING "GROSS"

Having a disease like CF does not make a person disgusting or "gross," but it can certainly feel that way at times. The preceding example about vomiting all over our bathroom from a combination of anesthesia and partial bowel obstruction offers as good an illustration as any. But perhaps the best example I can offer of this phenomenon in my own life comes from the time I lost control of my bowels in my spouse's car after a different surgery. If you know much about CF, you likely know that the bowel movements of most patients have some characteristic features in common. Specifically, the feces of people with CF tend to be both extremely oily (because of poor fat absorption) and extremely sticky (because of poor protein absorption). This makes them somewhat more difficult to clean up even in an ideal scenario.

Losing bowel control in the passenger seat of my spouse's car while still heavily sedated was distinctly not ideal. Yet she sanguinely cleaned up the mess and gave the upholstery on the seat a good scrubbing after making sure I took my next dose of antibiotics and got safely into bed to sleep off the anesthesia. The next day, I asked if I had done anything strange while still under sedation. My spouse mentioned a minor bowel accident but seemed unperturbed. I figured she meant I had a bit of leakage on my underwear. I did not learn the full extent of what had transpired until months later, during a moment where I felt more down about my body and my fitness as a sexual partner. She pointedly told me that I was always "the sexiest person [she knew], even when [I was] shitting in [her] car" and encouraged me to remember that her affection for me includes my CF. These days, that feels easier to remember.

The idea of "grossness" in living and aging with CF invokes both general impressions of the appearance of the body and specific elements of the mechanics of the body. A previous relationship partner once described me as a "disgusting skeleton" because the progressively worse pancreatic insufficiency I was dealing with caused me to lose additional weight in my early twenties and never regain it. I wrote about this a bit in "You Poor Thing," reflecting on that former partner's suggestion that I was somehow lucky to be with him because I was sick (Nowakowski 2016b). He explicitly told me that other people would not find me sexy or desirable. Of course, this same relationship also involved copious demonstrations of jealousy when other male-looking people would show interest in me. So, although the perception of bodily "grossness" played a pivotal role in this person's responses to me as a sexual being, it did so as part of a broader context of systemic inequality.

In "You Poor Thing" I described an encounter in which I was desperately looking for a bathroom at a major airport. Someone offered to help me find my gate, and behaved flirtatiously while doing so. But when they found out I was sick and urgently in need of toilet access, they immediately screwed up their face in disgust. The way their perception of my sexuality changed dramatically after I provided information about living with a chronic disease that affected my intestines illustrates a similar intersection of stigmas (Nowakowski 2016b). Envisioning the dynamics of chronic bowel issues likely played a strong role in the reaction of that individual upon learning why I actually appeared distressed. The person's initial apparent perception of me as a sex object also speaks to broader marginalization of female-looking bodies and the people who occupy them.

I recently read a delightfully familiar account of similar dynamics in long-term relationships with CF patients in a blog post from the girlfriend of one of my friends and fellow advocates, Gunnar Esiason. I have always enjoyed Gunnar's blog for its candid, good-humored, and remarkably upbeat discussion of topics often perceived as "taboo" in chronic illness management. Gunnar had shared previously on his blog about his relationship with his girlfriend Darcy Cunningham, and her increasing involvement in CF advocacy. He eventually invited Darcy to do a blog post of her own, which she focused on the "gross" elements of CF bodies and how intimate partners become acclimated to these things with time. She called the post "Gunnar Is Gross" but then proceeded to describe how things that seem unsettling can also be completely normal, and an important part of closeness with one's partner. In other words, Darcy demonstrated how things that initially seem "gross" can become a source of familiarity and bonding while still never losing their inherent sophomoric humor. Darcy's words proved very resonant for me and my spouse in a number of ways—the comfort with "squicky" topics, the gentle good humor, the sense of pride in really getting to know the full scope of someone's experiences as part of intimacy with them. Yet we also noted how these experiences are situated in Gunnar and Darcy's unique context as a straight-passing couple. I reflect in depth on these nuances in the discussion of situated sexuality later in the chapter.

Darcy's insightful blog post also illustrates how bowel issues tend to be a flashpoint for discourse on what is "gross" about inhabiting our CF bodies. Yet these kinds of challenges represent just one cluster of factors that may impact the sex lives of people living and aging with CF. Additional issues may include, but are certainly not limited to: sudden vomiting, mucus plugs, bleeding episodes, coughing fits, membrane tears, urine leakage, and joint grinding. I have experienced all of these at one point or another. Two stories stand out among the crowd, however. I recall vividly one instance of coughing up something that actually looked like a garden slug on my spouse's genitals while performing oral sex on her. We both laughed, disposed of the interloping mucus clot, and continued on as before. Although the experience felt momentarily awkward because it required pausing our intimacy to clean up the mucus plug, it also felt both extremely normal and hilariously funny. And the affection shining in my spouse's eyes at that shared moment of humor had emotional value all its own.

I also recall with equal clarity having to interrupt a tranquil moment of cuddling with another partner after vaginal intercourse to race to the bathroom. Rather than needing to empty my bowels, I had felt a sudden rush of moisture in my vaginal canal that I knew could not possibly be cervical mucus. The moment I bore down with my pelvic muscles, an impressive amount of blood shot out into the toilet. My initial surprised gasp quickly dissolved into peals of laughter. After verifying that I was okay, my partner rolled his eyes and said "nice job, GWAR," in reference to the macabre stage antics of a shock-metal band we both enjoyed.

Sex with CF thus implicates a variety of potential "gross" experiences that may arise without warning. Adapting to the normalcy of these experiences—and how they may become more severe with time as the disease continues to weather the body—constitutes an important part of achieving healthy sexuality in aging with CF. Of course, the concept of what constitutes a "normal" body in appearance or functioning varies dramatically according to social and cultural context. I was raised at a medical school where my parents taught neuroscience and—ironically enough—gross anatomy. I saw cadaver parts, both human and otherwise, on a regular basis. And beneath the fume hood in my parents' lab, I regularly saw the various internal organs and bodily secretions of euthanized mice being dissected for analysis. This kind of use of non-human animals made me uncomfortable and raised a lot of questions about consent and the greater good. However, it also gave me a deep familiarity with death itself, and with all the various "gross" things the body may produce while still alive. So, I thought little of experiences like urinating in "a dainty gingham-topped jam jar" and holding the sample up to the light for my parents to examine (Nowakowski 2017). I imagine this basic level of comfort with the macabre has continued to shape my reactions to such incidents. After all, how could I grow up in that kind of environment and not become at least somewhat hardcore?

Some people with CF adapt more easily than others to the progressively greater antagonism to which the disease subjects us and our partners as we continue to age. Social and cultural norms about bodies in a general sense, and aging bodies in a specific one, can absolutely impact individual people's experiences with health and illness transformation in sexuality and intimacy as the disease progresses. These norms can also intersect with other social locations and identities, and their implications for perceptions of sexual normalcy. For example, my queer identity may shape the ease with which I reconcile experiences of "grossness" with perceptions of myself as a sexual being. Indeed, public discourse on queer sexuality often implicates anal intercourse in the framing of queer intimacy as somehow dirty. Although this particular group of sexual activities may also feature prominently in the lives of heterosexual partners, it gets narrated socially as somehow unique to and defining of queerness.

My experiences of progressively adapting to a healthy sense of my own sexuality as a person aging with CF are indeed situated within the context of both a queer marriage and other partnerships that pass more effectively as straight. These experiences also speak to direct connections between the "gross" consequences of the disease and physical intimacy itself. Indeed, in some situations the physical challenges of living with CF actually invite greater bodily intimacy. I wrote about this briefly in a prior book chapter called "Death Check" in which I described the simultaneous horror and sweetness of my spouse having to clap me on the back for several minutes at a time just so I could cough out enough lurid green sludge to breathe (Nowakowski 2017). She would later tell me that helping me breathe at night was one of the most meaningful and special experiences of her life. Likewise, another partner teared up when I asked him to perform that same kind of percussive therapy on my back. He later noted that the invitation resonated clearly as an expression of trust and thus a welcoming into greater intimacy with me—both physically and beyond. And when I would present with symptoms of active pulmonary infection and not feel inclined to engage in explicitly sexual activity, he voiced aloud how much he treasured the physical connection of helping me cough up the infected mucus.

BUGS AS BEDFELLOWS

My spouse and I bonded quickly over many things the year we met, among them our shared interest in grunge music and specifically the band Pearl Jam.

We differed somewhat on our choice of favorite albums, and these differences often reflected the nuances of our personal biographies. My own favorite album unsurprisingly remains *Vitalogy*, whose music and artwork strongly engage concepts of embodiment and sexuality as manifestations of the macabre in everyday life. The album includes a delightfully whimsical track called "Bugs" in which Eddie Vedder explores uncertainty about whether to eschew or join forces with the bugs in his room. The loose wording lends itself to interpretation through multiple lenses. For me, this song has always evoked the recurrent infections I deal with—not only in my lungs, but also in other mucosa like my genital membranes. So, although I may not have bugs in my room, I definitely have them in many other private spaces.

Infections and the importance of constant preventive measures constitutes a prominent leitmotif in the sex lives of people living and aging with CF. It is entirely too easy for members of our patient community to get persistent infections—especially bacterial and fungal ones—in the genital and urinary mucosa. This can happen from time to time even if we do practice safe sex. It also falls to each of us to figure out what makes sexual activity as safe as possible for us as individual patients with particular embodiment and socialization contexts. And the costs of unsafe sexual activity can be shatteringly high, all the more so as we grow older and our bodies become more vulnerable to colonization by unfriendly organisms.

As a clinical educator in geriatrics, I routinely hear the advice that providers should not go looking for infections in patients of very advanced age, because they will find them. This perception admittedly has some truth to it. For example, a subclinical population of unfriendly bacteria in the intestine of an otherwise healthy eighty-five year old likely does not present cause for concern. However, a subclinical population of *Pseudomonas aeruguinosa* or *Escheria coli* traveling up the urethra and eventually taking root in the bladder, ureter, and kidneys of a thirty-five-year-old CF patient absolutely does (Nowakowski 2018a). Nothing ever seems to stay subclinical for long with us, which makes preventing infections before they start vitally important for healthy sexuality and sustainable aging (Nowakowski 2018b).

I have unfortunately become a case in point of this essential truth about progressive disease. When various virulent infections in my genital and urinary mucosa were not addressed in time to halt their progression up into my renal system from my urinary tract, I paid the price in kidney damage that would never be reversed, along with substantial suffering in the shorter term. Pyelonephritis, a syndrome associated with infection in the kidneys, causes both terrible pain and substantial impacts to the body's physical appearance. It also saps energy and greatly reduces quality of life. So far, I have experienced prolonged bouts of pyelonephritis due to *Pseudomonas aeruguinosa*, *Escheria coli*, and *Staphyloccus aureus*. And I now live with chronic kidney disease that, although well managed, will never go away (Nowakowski 2018a).

This story has a qualified happy ending—something commonplace in tales of aging with CF. Because my care team and I now possess greater understanding of what safe sex means for me, I am able to take consistent preventive measures to keep my renal and genitourinary systems as healthy as possible. These include urinating both before and after any kind of sexual activity, wiping down my genitals and my partner's thoroughly before and after any kind of intercourse, applying copious lubricant before any type of penetration, using condoms in any instance where a partner may wish to ejaculate in contact with my genital mucosa, washing and sanitizing hands regularly, using medications like d-mannose to prevent bacterial colonization in the urinary and renal mucosa, and maintaining strict rules against close contact between my partners and anyone else who has CF. Making these instrumental changes in my self-management has also required cognitive changes in my relationship with self and others. Specifically, I have had to adapt to changing notions of what constitutes "sexiness" in behavioral practice.

This ongoing process involves questioning normative concepts of enjoyment, and specifically the idea that measures to protect my health might make sexual activity "no fun." Lived experience of past relationships—and in some cases abuse—opened my eyes early and often to the idea that some people would find my health challenges burdensome. I have heard people describe my desire not to be in pain or wind up with an infection in various derogatory ways. The term "mood killer" has been used to describe the somber note that being reminded of my mortality introduces into intimacy. My basic protective measures like urinating and washing before and after intercourse have been framed as "unromantic" for interrupting the "natural flow" of sex. I have also heard my desire to protect myself from serious infections described as "TMI." How anything could constitute an excess of private information when one person is about to insert their body into another's still boggles my mind.

I suspect that what people were actually saying in that regard was that they perceived my body as somehow disgusting, and perhaps even taboo because of it. This again evokes the perception of "grossness" in the CF body, but also deeply rooted individual cultural fears of serious illness and eventual death. The same partners who reacted adversely to my actions in protection of my own health were those who stated explicitly that they would "have to think about" hanging around if I were to become considerably sicker. One of those individuals would later go on to abandon me in the intensive care unit. This experience felt impossibly lonely in the moment, but over time became an exceptionally valuable lesson about what really constitutes "safety" in a relationship. And perhaps the constant looming specter of deadly infection also evokes a certain discomfort with death itself. After all, mortality is hardly unique to people with CF, just more omnipresent and examined from a young age.

Reckoning with our own mortality is a constant with CF from the time we first learn we have the disease. Sometimes this awareness comes earlier still in those of us whose conclusive diagnoses took longer in coming despite being preceded by many years of serious health problems. We grow comfortable with death as yet another strange bedfellow in addition to all those bugs. We understand the possibility of bargaining with death for a little more time in a little better health—a prospect that grows more realistic with every passing year. As I write an early draft of this chapter, the press release announcing the submission for FDA approval of Vertex's new "triple combo" of CFTR modulator drugs for broad-spectrum treatment of multiple classes of gene mutations is only hours old. As an aside, I find it difficult to describe in a few words the immense promise of something like the triple combo. In the CF community, we become so steeped in vast quantities of technical terminology that we often wind up code switching between disease-specific spaces and more general ones. I see this pattern reflected in the communications of friends and colleagues with other chronic conditions. But a particular feature of CF remains that constant reckoning with the prospect of early mortality preceded by a long period of suffering. That enduring process makes you hardcore from a very young age—and may also instill a certain pride in this toughness as described in the next section.

People with CF grow accustomed to living with diverse and profound challenges in our own daily lives. Infections and the need to prevent them constitute one group of daily challenges that impact areas of our lives not directly related to CF. Perhaps because of this, we often feel much more aware and self-conscious of those things when building intimacy with others. This may occur because the process of growing close to others makes us wrestle with cognitive dissonance. The contrast between normative ideas about enjoyable relationships and intimacy and the reality of what we must do to keep ourselves safe in sexual activity can frankly feel like whiplash even after years of experience. So, the pursuit of safe sex with CF introduces a dichotomy of being hardcore and being vulnerable that characterizes the experience of intimacy within our broader journey of lifelong illness management. Perhaps this explains why we often regard our community elders as almost legendary figures of toughness, veritable gladiators matched against nothing so much as our own traitorous bodies.

INJURIES, PAIN, AND TOUGHNESS

Conceptualizing the fight to stay well with CF as an arena battle of sorts seems remarkably apt, even in cases where people prefer the softer side of sexual activity. The constant threat of pain and injury looms eternally in my mind no matter how much I might be enjoying a given encounter. Certain types of sexual activity are tricky propositions for me even on the best of days where my mucus is comparatively thinner and my bacterial loads are comparatively lower. My history of sexual abuse also includes internal injuries that led to scarring and rigidity in the vaginal and cervical tissue. With these physical challenges as well as more intangible complications of past abuse, sexual activity itself also becomes quixotic on a broader level. Performing toughness has different nuances across these contexts for me and others with CF who reckon with similar history in their own lives.

Likewise, each of us performs toughness differently in our sexual relationships and deals with adverse events in our own unique ways. Some people respond to injuries or other evidence of physical trauma by withdrawing or dissociating. I did this at certain times in the past, but increasingly preferred to "lean in" to physical problems and master the situation through macabre humor. A "hardcore" response to injury or the evidence of same (like the infamous "GWAR" incident with vaginal bleeding after intercourse) generally supersedes other actions when something goes wrong. However, this almost hypermasculine dismissal of any horror I might feel both intertwines and contrasts with the constant vigilance about when pain might begin or when an injury might occur. No matter how comfortable I might feel in the moment during a given sexual encounter, I can never fully dispel the consciousness of how it might go wrong—and of how I might pay dearly for those outcomes. Yet as with life in general, perhaps this instills in me a greater appreciation for the pleasure I find in sexual intimacy, and especially in forms of intercourse that once evoked strong associations with abuse.

In "The Salt Without the Girl" I devoted ample attention to the performance of masculinity as both an authentic expression of self and a means of coping with the brutality of progressive disease (Nowakowski 2019b). Yet as an agender person, my experiences of gendered embodiment both invoke and transcend constructions of "tough" masculinity. My behaviors both within and outside of intimate relationships involve elements of both masculinities and femininities. I often engage diverse presentations of both masculinity and femininity in tandem while framing these performances as outside the realm of affirming a specifically gendered self. I also access parts of myself that appear more masculine or more feminine to others differently in the varied social spaces where I spend time. This includes my intimate relationships, which tend to be plural as my spouse and I have always practiced consensual nonmonogamy (Sumerau and Nowakowski 2019).

Although I have a cohesive self-concept, I experience my body and its impacts from CF differently within one of my present relationships versus the other. In my marriage, I quite reliably embody the butch lesbian trope of the "stone top." This archetype involves strongly masculine behavior during both sex and other types of interactions. Yet it also provides something of a cover for any awkwardness I might feel about taking time to prevent transmission of bacteria or other unfriendly organisms. I never need this cover in my marriage; my spouse reminds me frequently she always finds me sexy and feels tremendous closeness with me. But interpreting my sexual persona in my marriage through a stone butch lens helps me feel better and more confident about myself. Because stone tops generally do not want their genitals touched in absence of an express request, I always know I can pause the action to wipe myself down or otherwise take preventive measures without somehow disrupting another person's exploration of my body. I also know that I can stop doing any given form of contact at any time without giving so much as a word of explanation, without either me or my spouse perceiving any loss of intimacy. Not only do I know this intellectually, but I also consistently embrace this knowledge affectively. And my balanced performance of toughness and watchfulness has gradually extended the intimacy of explicitly sexual contact well beyond those boundaries in my marriage. My spouse frequently remarks that she "[feels] like we are always having sex" because of how intimate every shared activity has become at this point in our shared journey.

In my other relationship, balancing my desire to perform toughness with my responsibility to protect my health requires more active engagement with my own sense of worth and the value of my own safety over any momentary feelings of emotional discomfort my partner might feel. Although he does not have the same level of closeness and trust with me that my spouse does, my other partner consistently prioritizes my comfort and well-being in all of our physical intimacy and enjoys participating actively in my CF management. However, I also access more feminine elements of my selfhood and my sexuality in that relationship in more overtly physical ways. I thus wrestle with feeling more acutely responsible for my partner's emotional state during sex. Reconciling this with my desire to prevent infections can prove challenging in the moment despite my overarching knowledge that this matters to my partner.

I also sometimes catch myself performing toughness in less constructive ways in my nonmarital relationship, both within and outside of sexual activity. The trope of the stoical woman who silently endures pain so as to protect others from its emotional and social consequences has proven more relevant in those spaces. Yet I have also begun to see the rewards of showing vulnerability as a means of affirming self and even creating closeness with others during physical intimacy. A particular memory of one encounter with my partner, during which I suddenly grimaced and said something hurt, stands out in my mind because of how he reacted. He immediately withdrew from my body and expressed compassion for my pain. And then, with an enormous grin and bright eyes, he wrapped me up in his arms and lay down beside me. I have often pointed to this encounter during conflicts in other areas of our relationship as evidence of his ability to cheerfully embrace whatever I am experiencing in the moment.

When toughness becomes an affectation as described above rather than an authentic performance, I reflect on the bigger question of whom my sexuality is actually for. By extension, I also explore the question of for whom I perform toughness within that context of sexuality as directed experience. Clearly, I do not owe any of my relationship partners a specific performance of gender identity, CF management, or the intersection of the two. Yet I also embrace the individuality of both my spouse and my partner, and understand that they may receive different messages from the same basic set of actions. I reflect actively on how to communicate affection and warmth while also being hardcore and keeping myself safe—a set of balls I continually juggle while also attempting to observe and critically reflect on each individually.

The pursuit of safe sex with CF thus involves a constant performance and reevaluation of what I call "situated toughness." This leads me to reflect on how sexual activity itself, whether with progressive disease or otherwise, is a profoundly situated experience. In my present relationships, I have ample space to explore these questions in both private reflection and shared dialogue. I also generally feel energized by the relationships themselves rather than exhausted and drained. Living with CF itself often proves immensely tiring. Yet I no longer find the usual bodily impacts of managing the disease weaponized against me as evidence of my inferiority in sexual partnership.

SEX AS SITUATED EXPERIENCE

In times gone by, I absolutely did find the consequences of my CF weaponized against me—all the more so because the disease had not yet been conclusively diagnosed. I wrote in "Death Check" about my simultaneous experiences with being told I was "faking it" and being maligned for not taking my illness "seriously enough." My spouse would later tell me that "the definition of abuse is a situation in which you can never win" no matter what you do. At the time, this understanding remained far removed from my daily life. I focused, as many people in similar circumstances do, on surviving. This meant, among other things, enduring the repeated violation of my body and the ways this injured me physically and mentally. Although my body was narrated as disgusting and undesirable, it was also framed as an object for the pleasure of another and treated accordingly. And like many other abuse survivors, I also experienced stigmatization about other social locations that intersected with my CF: my Polish and Tuscarora heritage, my family's class background, my pursuit of graduate education. It was perhaps telling that I got denigrated for having both disadvantage in some forms and privilege in others.

Some memories from those years swirl together in an indistinct blur of sorrow; others pierce through with vivid clarity. I remember sitting in bathtubs, doubled over in pain and bleeding from my vaginal canal, and then trying later to clean the injured membranes gently with diluted peroxide so infection would not set in. All of this hurt. I also learned quickly that I was not to leave any evidence of blood. And if I spent too long in the bathroom, meticulously cleaning countertops and the rims of toilets, the door would begin to shake from pounding fists. The words "what are you doing in there" still haunt me. Sometimes no amount of locked doors between me and the rest of the world makes me feel completely safe. Clearing my larynx in the bathroom sink, I run the tap endlessly, afraid to leave any trace of bloody cement on the ceramic. During vaginal intercourse, I like to place dark towels beneath my body. The deeper colors soften the appearance of infected mucus and mute the grayish red hue of blood from ruptured vessels. And I still fear, seeing a partner withdraw from my body, their potential reaction to traces of blood or thick clots of mucus on the outside of a condom. But I look—I always look. After all, I am no coward.

A great irony of all this was that I always took my illness seriously enough to examine every bit of evidence of how it was devastating my body and my prospects for a future. And if I faked anything, it was the appearance of being well—of functioning normally or having things under control. I entered the ICU with a serum potassium of 2.1 milliequivalents per liter, my field of vision narrowed to a dark tunnel and my heartbeat barely clinging to its rhythm. Death should have found me ages before that point. What does "safe sex" even mean when you have both feet dangling into an early grave? I had no energy to contemplate this then, let alone desire. This too became weaponized against me. I cringe every time I hear the word "frigid" even when it is only used in reference to temperature.

I would later do some research on this as well—the simultaneous desexualization and resentment of people with chronic conditions whose desire declines (Nowakowski and Sumerau 2019b). Along with my spouse and a colleague, I used some survey data to explore relationships between inflammatory diseases, biomarkers of swelling, and feeling obligated to have sex. We found that diagnosed inflammatory conditions correlated with reduced perceptions of pressure to have sex. However, we did not find the same pattern for biomarker evidence of inflammation, despite higher levels of these biomarkers also being associated with more unpleasant experiences during sex such as pain. We thus found further evidence for reification of diagnosed specific disease as the only legitimate reason for reduced sexual activity related to illness, even among our oldest participants. This research and other studies using the same dataset challenged a variety of misconceptions about people becoming nonsexual as part of usual aging. It also showed nuances in the social and behavioral expectations of people with different types of chronic conditions as they age.

The research on inflammatory diseases and perceived sexual obligation offered a specific view of a much broader and more widespread phenomenon documented in the health and aging literature. Not surprisingly, our findings for those studies differed heavily along sex lines. Participants who identified as male rarely experienced any feelings of obligation to have sex. By contrast, these experiences proved common among participants identifying as female. We also reflected on how generational culture likely played a role in the socialization of participants, who were all fifty-seven or older in 2005. Available evidence suggested that gender role socialization shaped people's sense of appropriate behavior within intimate partnerships (see also Harder and Sumerau 2019). In those articles and others, we also noted a pressing need for greater attention to older women's sexual health in general and sexual health specifically (Nowakowski and Sumerau 2019c). We joined other colleagues in interdisciplinary geriatrics research in calling for creative, diverse amplification of the experiences of women, femmes, and females aging with a variety of different health conditions. And we situated this inquiry in a broader call for bringing scholarship on chronic illness within relationships "out of the shadow" to include partnerships with multiple people living with health conditions (Nowakowski and Sumerau 2017a). Exploring the evolution of safe sex across the life course among people with CF represents one thread in a vast tapestry of possible inquiry on this topic.

Evolving understanding and practice of safe sex in aging with CF also necessarily invokes broader metaphysical questions about the nature of sexual activity itself, and its relationship to intimacy. Sexual activity is a broad category of ways of sharing closeness with other people. It is also a social and cultural construct that intertwines with other sources of meaning in our lives. Among people living and aging with progressive diseases, sexual activity can take on nuances unique to changes in physical and cognitive functioning over the natural course of an illness (Nowakowski and Sumerau 2017b). It can remain a profound celebration of life and vitality, even as health status dramatically worsens. It can also offer a means of reckoning with death on the journey through disease. I have often reflected that French speakers describe orgasms as *petites mortes* for reasons well beyond poetic license. The experience of liberation from the body, however briefly it lasts before corporeality sets back in with startling ferocity, truly does offer a feeling of transcendence. And how we achieve that feeling of ethereality as we age can evolve dynamically.

It will thus come as little surprise that I am presently working with another colleague on a book called *Sexual Deviance in Health and Aging* (Ritter and Nowakowski forthcoming). Rather than treating illness as an afterthought in the exploration of human sexuality and its intersection with social norms, this book places chronic disease centrally within a broad ecology of human sexual biography. Core threads in the book also include queer sexuality, nonbinary gender experience, and consensual nonmonogamy. And we devote an entire chapter to dynamic shifts in the meaning of sex as people continue to age—as well as the intersection of these shifts with generational norms and shifting cultural mores about the moral and ethical dimensions of sexual contact. In all cases, sex remains a profoundly situated construct, with respect to chronology as much as anything else.

CONCLUDING REFLECTIONS

So . . . what does it mean to be sexual with CF? I suppose I am still figuring that out for myself, day by day. My reflections on personal experience and prior literature illustrate the deeply situated and nuanced nature of sexuality in aging with progressive disease. I often find myself wondering how my present experiences of safe and healthy sexuality with CF might differ from where I have been in the past, and from where I will go as I continue to age. But with the benefit of some hindsight already, I can certainly predict a few things for the future. I make meaning surrounding safe sex first and foremost by being "hardcore of a different kind." I coined this phrase in jest while relaxing with my spouse on our living room couch one evening. That couch has served as the point of origin for many of my best ideas in scholarship and outreach. But the idea of being hardcore in a special sort of way also spoke to me on a deeper level, beyond the winking reference to pornography and the potential for a snappy line or two. It illustrated how my personality played into my sexuality and defined it, both with the parameters of and well beyond my experiences with CF itself.

These reflections have thus led me to wonder how this meaning-making surrounding CF and sexuality may differ for me and for others or remain the same depending on circumstance. I turn back, as I often do, to Ian Pettigrew's wonderful *Salty Girls* photo series and Andy Lipman's uplifting *CF Warrior Project* book. I never participated in *Salty Girls* directly, but I absolutely found inspiration in the ways each model shared her sexual self with the camera—sometimes boldly, sometimes chastely, always uniquely. *Salty Girls* both celebrates the sexual power of people living with CF and encourages viewers to look well beyond it. This process of looking beyond came into sharp focus for me as a participant in the *CF Warrior Project* book, which condensed the ambitions and achievements of sixty-five different adults with CF into brief profiles. Sexuality was not a core emphasis of the book, yet it appeared as informal curriculum in many of the stories when the final version went to press. For example, the book shares tales of people expanding their families, or living their truth in queer love. In different ways, *Salty Girls* and the *CF Warrior Project* book show how being hardcore pervades every aspect of sexuality with CF—from the recreational to the professional to the reproductive.

In an age where CF care and thus longevity are improving rapidly, notions of dynamic sexuality across the life course absolutely impact our understanding of what it means to live and age with CF. This dialogue pervades many community spaces, including the CF specific Facebook groups in which I participate and breakout sessions at Cystic Fibrosis Foundation conference events. Being hardcore appears as a common theme, although not always in those precise words. Stories about coughing up mucus plugs on a partner, having random lung or genital bleeds during intercourse, losing bowel control, staining sheets with the oily residue of steatorrhea, or vomiting because of an obstruction all show up with some regularity. And the stories often seem to grow gorier and more explicit with posters' increasing age.

As we progress through life while holding the murderous beast within us at bay, we become more accustomed to the indignities with which it subjects us. In sexuality as in other areas, we achieve dominion over the beast by hardening ourselves against its horrors—a sort of beating the enemy at its own game. When we become fortunate enough to reach midlife or beyond, we begin to understand how little separation exists between celebrating life and laughing at the evidence of incipient death.

Yet perhaps paradoxically, our chances of continuing to stave off death depend on exercising caution even as we cultivate notions of hardcore toughness. CF hardly stands out from other progressive conditions in this regard, although it has some particular nuances that make for especially compelling stories about macabre moments in bed. Amplifying specific stories of balancing our hardcore emotional mastery of the fear involved in living with CF with our mindful cultivation of sexual wellness through safe practice offers value for further research on healthy aging.

First, it highlights opportunities for broader exploration of sexuality across the life course in populations often not considered sexual in prior inquiry. Second, it demands examination of mechanisms for supporting sexual wellness in intersectionally marginalized populations as they age. Third, it invites investigation of how progressive disease may impact the meaning and nature of sexuality as people live longer with such conditions. Fourth, it illuminates how sexuality can become a tool for mastery of chronic disease itself. Suffice it to say that the legendary Bob Flanagan would be proud.

Chapter Two

Rejecting Simplicity in Favor of Embracing the Complexity of Multifaceted Health and Aging

When I first sat down to write this chapter, I immediately thought about two things. First, I thought about just how much my life changed for the better as a result of going to graduate school, and in so doing, developing a successful career as a sociological social psychologist and novelist writing about inter-sections of sexualities, gender, health, religion, and violence in society. However, the second thing that I thought about was the way that contemporary social norms surrounding health and healthcare access almost kept me out of graduate school in the first place. It is remarkably easy to demarcate my life in terms of my life before and my life after gaining access to a steady paycheck and supportive social networks through my graduate school experience. At the same time, it is just as easy to remember how close I came to being turned away from this path before it began.

I remember this, what would become pivotal, moment in my life as if it was yesterday. I was standing in a shack that served as an apartment I could afford. I was watching one of the many roaches who shared the residence scurry across the floor. I was looking over the necessary paperwork for graduate school, and what I needed to do to start the program that fall. I was drinking water that was a bit gray but was also free from the rusty tap in the apartment style shack. There was pain radiating through my face from inju-ries I would get surgically repaired nine years later when I could finally afford to do so both financially and emotionally. I was excited about going to graduate school. I was thrilled that the graduate program funding package would pay me more than any job I had gained to that point in my life (i.e., about $14,000 per year). I was trying to figure out if I had enough spare cash to eat that day, or if I would be better off waiting until the next day when there would be an event on my college campus with free food. I was too excited for this to bother me, and that alone was a nice change.

Unfortunately, my excitement faded in a heartbeat when I got to the point in the paperwork that told me I would need health insurance to begin the graduate program. I also knew that the cheapest option for health insurance provided by the university I was about to attend was about $1,600.00 more than I had in the bank. I also already knew, from curiosity about fixing my face, that this was my cheapest option if I had to have health insurance. I already knew I didn't have any credit. I just had a job that paid by the hour. I knew that wasn't enough. My job at the time paid me what I considered a great wage at the time because it was more than most of the wages I had ever had, but it was still only about eight bucks an hour and it left me with just enough—plus student loans during undergraduate semesters and the occasional commission from writing for local newspapers and magazines—to squeak by on bills, eat at least every other day, and occasionally go have discount beers or pizza slices with friends if I budgeted everything to the last cent.

I looked at the paperwork, thought about the money I did not have for the insurance I did not have, and thought about the gun I found in the apartment the previous year and kept for no particular reason. A shot of pain went through my face about the same time my stomach seemed to scream at me for food I did not have available for it at the time. I had already long decided I was getting out of the life I had lived up until that point, and if health insurance meant no graduate school, then I wondered if maybe I should consider other options. I picked up a pack of stale cigarettes on the top of the rusty refrigerator, changed from my inside the house protect my feet from the roaches shoes (i.e., a pair of closed toe slippers with thick soles) to my outside the house shoes (i.e., six year old at the time sneakers), and walked outside. I stood outside chain smoking stale cigarettes for a couple hours cursing and crying.

I went through a few different options over the next couple months. I had time, and I looked at my options the same way any other intelligent college graduate might. I also had access to the computer lab at my undergraduate college, which gave me access to the internet even when the internet wasn't working that well at the coffee shop downtown. I considered going on the road with a friend who had a gig with contractors building houses and doing other construction work across the Midwest. I considered paying a guy in Swansea, South Carolina, who was known to be able to create and back up fake documentation for things like health, car, and other types of insurance that folks needed to show proof of for jobs, homes, and other necessities that are anything but guaranteed in the United States. I still don't know if that guy really existed or if it was a myth because I finally, after weeks in the computer lab at my now alma mater, made two discoveries. First, there was a part of the health insurance requirement, in the fine print, that noted it could be paid as part of school fees, and therefore, one could use student loans to cover it. Second, there was the decision to take out student loans to make health insurance and thus graduate school possible even though the original plan had been to be finished taking out loans after finishing my undergraduate education.

As I write this chapter now, I think about the contradiction in the experiences shared above. On the one hand, universities often require students to have health insurance to attend classes, and this is said to be an effort to improve the health of students and the campus community. On the other hand, this requirement may require some non-traditional students from lower economic classes to take on more debt to attend school, which both limits how much school may improve their economic standing and creates stress likely to negatively impact their health over time as they navigate debt they were required to obtain in the name of the health of others. This contradiction, that one should pursue things that might improve their health and well-being but doing so may require one to do unhealthy things, is always in the forefront of my mind when I think about health in the United States and in my life. It is especially relevant when I think about the ways sex, gender, sexualities, class, and other social locations intersect in my own and others' experiences of health and aging.

In this chapter, I thus explore contradictions in health and aging that become visible and relevant when one does not fit into normative assumptions about sex, gender, sexualities, class, and other socio-demographic locations. In so doing, I seek to highlight the ways "health" itself is a contextual term that can mean many different things depending upon the other aspects of one's life, and the ways those other aspects limit or expand opportunities for managing both health and aging on the one hand, and surviving life in a society where one occupies marginalized social locations on the other. To this end, I utilize my experiences as a non-binary, bisexual, poly trans woman who has moved from the lower-working to the upper middle class in the past decade to illuminate and problematize contradictory notions of what we mean when we say "health" or "well-being" in relation to broader social norms and inequalities in the United States at present.

AM I HEALTHY?

I have to be honest here. I honestly do not know if I am healthy. The truth is that existing literature in public health, medical sociology, medical science, biology, and other fields is not all that helpful in answering this question for me. The truth is that the answer is likely that I am both healthy and unhealthy in a wide variety of ways depending on how any given authority might demarcate what counts as membership in either of these categories. In its simplest form, I would likely say that I am healthy enough as I feel good most of the time, and my body and mind function well enough for me to handle most of the tasks I would like to or need to handle in the ongoing experience of my personal and professional life. If, however, I attempt to more clearly situate myself into any given set of health models, things become much more complicated.

There are, for example, many ways in which I would likely appear at least as or even far healthier than the average person in the United States. Specifically, I have great health insurance, and access to many different aspects of healthcare, healthcare systems, and specialists should the need arise. Likewise, I exercise regularly, eat well, monitor and maintain solid nutrition, consume more than enough clean water on a daily basis, possess work that is both challenging and rewarding mentally and emotionally, and have a powerful network of social support I can draw on at any time for any reason. Further, I have a spouse, the first author of this book, who is a medical expert personally and professionally, and who is connected to a network of other medical professionals through both their own career and their management of cystic fibrosis (see chapter 1 for more information). Finally, I have, thus far, a rather strong immune system and very rarely get sick beyond seasonal and environmental colds and other minor ailments from time to time. By many approximations of what it means to be "healthy," these characteristics would find me at or near the optimal models of health and aging for a middle-aged person.

At the same time, however, there are other ways I would appear far less than healthy or just plain unhealthy based on existing models of health and aging. Specifically, I manage and negotiate chronic pain in my back, legs, and feet due to violence and incidental injuries suffered at earlier points in my life. Likewise, I continue to smoke cigarettes on most days, drink socially and even more so at times when I feel especially stressed, and due to nightmares and other residue from past trauma, I have never developed any of what existing models would consider a consistent, healthy pattern of sleeping over time. Further, I spent over a decade heavily using Ibuprofen and other over-the-counter and prescription pain killers to manage injuries in my face I could not afford to fix in a more productive manner, and these efforts may someday come back to haunt my kidneys, liver, or other organ function, though that does not as yet appear to be the case. Finally, I avoid medical professionals as much as possible as a result of negative experiences with them in my youth and early twenties, and as a result, I am not yet fully claiming the benefits of my current possession of access to quality healthcare at this stage in my life. As such, one could pull any of these aspects of my life, and then they could argue that I would fit into models for less than ideal or even poor health and aging for a middle-aged person.

My case thus represents an example of the complexities and contradictions of singular conceptualization of what constitutes health (Sanders, Antin, Hunt, and Young 2019). Put simply, most health models in the contemporary United States seek to postulate a singular, linear path wherein some things are deemed healthy and normal, and others are deemed unhealthy and abnormal (see also Johnson 2015; Nowakowski and Sumerau 2019b; Sumerau and Mathers 2019). In so doing, however, medical authorities simplify the complexity, contradictions, and nuances of lived experience, and in so doing, limit what may or may not be considered healthy for a given people or group of persons in relation to the specific context of their own lives, social locations, and possibilities for health access and care (see also Samuels 2014). As such, whether or not I am healthy depends on which linear, simplified model I look at, and thus means that ultimately it depends on which, if any, model I am willing to put my own trust in as a human. This is why I honestly do not know whether or not I am healthy.

Let us Talk about Sex, Gender, and Sexualities Now

As readers are likely already well aware of at this point in this book, these dynamics—am I healthy—become even more complicated when we consider sex, gender, and sexualities. In the case of sex, for example, I have always felt female and interpreted and reacted to my body as a female one even though I was assigned male at birth. This has meant at least three things for the development of my own health and aging over time. First, my understanding of myself as a female led me to tuck and otherwise physically adjust parts of my body, especially after puberty, in ways that I didn't know at the time could create damage to my genital areas, and that at present, have led to a situation where I have some bruising, scarring, and sensitivity in these areas (see also Pearce 2018 for discussions of trans health more broadly). Second, my desire to make my body look more like other types of females (i.e., the ones others would be assigned as such in a doctor's office, for example) led me to pursue and use off-market hormones at times earlier in my life, and there is no way to know what, if any, long-term effects these may have had on my body (see also Johnson 2015 for discussions of social pressure to appear as others define one should appear in terms of gender). Finally, my ongoing desire to potentially further and even fully transition my body into one more conventionally defined as female continues to be a source of incredible stress, fear, and frustration for me as I continue to age (see Sumerau and Mathers 2019 for other examples of trans women navigating such feelings). In each of these ways, I don't know if I would be healthy or not in comparison to other trans, cis, or other types of women because there are not health models to answer this question.

Of course, as I've written elsewhere (Sumerau 2020; 2019), these sex experiences also influence my experience of gender, and thus the ways gender impacts my own health and aging as a body, personality, and otherwise. Although I always considered myself a woman and sought to transition so much so that I was willing to use off-market hormones, I also chose to put these feelings on hold, to an extent, to attempt to get out of the lower-working class through the pursuit of college and then graduate education. This meant that for multiple years I lived three separate lives most of the time (see, e.g., Goffman 1959; 1963; 1977 for navigating multiple selves in one body). In one life, I was the professional, quiet, shy, feminine person who seemed to be an effeminate guy to many people, and worked as hard or harder than others to succeed. In the next life, I was the lover and friend who was more feminine in private than in public and who privately said they were non-binary or trans feminine until finishing graduate school and then publicly said they were non-binary with the comfort of a decent salary. In the third life, I was myself—a female misdiagnosed as male who was a woman named Janis Erica but who kept herself secret and only became herself in private when no one—not even friends, lovers, or other close contacts—was around throughout graduate school, allowed some close loved ones to know this aspect of myself once I had a good job and some security, and more recently began to be more publicly open about who I am now that I have more economic security.

In fact, there were only three people I shared my true experience of myself with until recently. This was because part of setting up these different lives involved cutting ties with almost everyone who knew certain versions of me before I entered college in my mid-twenties and remaining mostly secret and quiet about myself throughout the years that followed. In 2012, however, I began to emotionally fall apart from carrying these multiple selves in isolation, and against my better judgement at the time, I reached out for help from my best friend, my then partner and now partner and spouse who is also the first author of this book, and my birth mother who was like a best friend to me from 2010 when we met for the first time since I was a baby until her death in 2014. Luckily for me, my better judgment at the time was incorrect, and these people became my closest confidants, and until 2017, when I began to be more open about who I am throughout my life, they were the secret source of support who knew all three lives I was living and aided such endeavors.

The scenario above suggests that one would need three different existing models of health and aging to understand my experiences for over a decade of my life as I pursued the educational credentials and career I have now. First, one might look to men's or masculine health models to understand my public persona in graduate school and at times later in my early years as a college professor (see Courtenay 2000 for discussion). Second, one might look to the very few emerging discussions of non-binary people's health to make sense of my private life in graduate school and more of my public life as a college professor over time (see Sumerau and Mathers 2019 for discussion). Third, one would look to the, again limited but emerging, models of trans women's lives to understand my secret life in graduate school, private life as a college professor before tenure, and currently becoming public life now (see again Sumerau and Mathers 2019 for discussion). In all three cases, how gender and health intertwine in my life become difficult to understand with existing health models that assume one gender identity in a life at any given time instead of potential multiple gender identities in multiple facets of life predicated upon what feels safe or available in certain contexts.

At the same time, sexualities always existed in the mixture of these three lives. This was both because openly bisexual and poly people are not common aspects of academic populations, and as mentors cautioned me before I entered graduate study and I saw for myself over time as well, not exactly welcome yet in such settings where monogamy and monosexuality remain almost entirely unquestioned and normative in both interpersonal interactions and scholarship (see also Barringer et al. 2018; Sumerau, Mathers, and Moon 2019; Sumerau 2019). As such, I continued to live and interact with others as a bi, pan, queer person and a poly person outside of academic contexts, but I downplayed these aspects of myself for the first few years while I gained graduate credentials and began to build my career. Over time, I then began to both write about and openly discuss and present these aspects of myself in my academic life (see Sumerau 2019 for example). As a result, however, this was another way that my own health trajectory would require multiple models to understand because, in some ways, my professional life was more like a closeted lesbian, gay, or bi person whereas my personal life was the opposite (see Adams 2011; Halkitis 2013; Schrock et al. 2014 for discussions of sexual minorities and health over the life course). Considering existing research demonstrates both of these conditions can impact health in many ways, my own experience raises questions about how both might play out together in the health of a single person.

As I've written about elsewhere (Sumerau 2017), these dynamics were further complicated as I began to process the trauma from being raped at a younger age while I was in graduate school living these multiple lives. Especially as I had never told anyone about those experiences at the time, I had never learned what, if any, lasting damage had been done to my body in the process (see Martin 2005 for discussion of physical and mental health effects tied to experiences of sexual violence). I also had no way of knowing what, if any, impact the injuries I had suffered to my face and other parts of my body due to other types of assaults I survived over time might have upon my aging and health over time. Since graduate school became the first time I felt like I had time to think, process, and slow down after years just trying to pay bills, manage the pain in my body and mind, and survive, my career development became intertwined with the necessity of managing past traumas, making sense of how these things influenced the rest of my life, and figuring out how to do these things while also building a career. As a result, sexualities—in terms of both identities and past negative experiences—became a common aspect of my life, trauma recovery processes, and negotiation as I aged.

The combination of the experiences above can be synthesized in the following insight—there are no current medical or health or aging scripts or models for those of us who must navigate multiple sex, gender, and sexual lives at the same time as a result of existing sex, gender, and sexual inequalities within society. Existing health and aging pathways generally assume one sex, gender, or sexual highway and even when they go beyond this assumption, they generally rely upon status passages and other bifurcated notions of before and after that again assume one is only aging or managing health as one thing at a given time. As such, they offer no way to understand or make sense of the contradictions and multiplicities illustrated by my experience. What might health, medicine, and other aspects of aging look like if we did consider more fluid possibilities in the lives—singular and plural—people live over time?

This question lies at the heart of the examples above. It also finds voice, to an extent, in each of the chapters of this book. What might happen to health and medicine if we opened up our minds to a multitude of options instead of seeking to create static, specific pathways and models? What might our understanding of—and potential empathy for—humanity look like if we sought to understand all the complexity, contradiction, and multiplicity instead of simplifying things into this model, that framework, or those statistical probabilities? Of course, this is an empirical question that could only be answered if we made such an attempt. Even so, however, for those of us who do not fit neatly into linear expectations or models, such answers may be the most likely way that we will ever have a chance at person-centered, quality healthcare (see also Nowakowski and Sumerau 2019a; Sanders et al. 2019).

Can We Talk about Class for a Minute?

At this point, it is important to note that each of the dynamics outlined above were dramatically shaped by the economic and social class locations wherein I experienced my early life as well as the rise in class status I have experienced in the past decade-plus. When I was twenty-seven years old, for example, the thought of finding a way to purchase this luxury named health insurance almost kept me from pursuing the educational and career path that led me out of the lower-working class. At the same time, the lower-working class shaped what little efforts I was able to make in terms of pursuing transition, life as a woman, and sexual practice long before I was writing about these things for a living. Further, my class status shaped the entirety of my graduate school experience as well as what my life looks like as a college professor at present in a wide variety of ways that may or may not be as easily noticeable to others. Put simply, nothing in this chapter, or anything related to health and aging more broadly (see Link and Phelan 1995), can be understood without also thinking about class as a social location.

This is especially important because I did not grow up at the very bottom of the economic structure of the United States. I was raised by adoptive parents who benefited, as so many white people did (see Gates 2013), from racialized labor and housing markets, and thus had solid, lower-working class jobs and the ability to own a decent home in a quiet southern neighborhood. Put simply, even as a child I didn't have the worst economic chances. As a result, the fact that the economic disadvantages I have faced so dramatically impacted my life both demonstrates the way social and economic class shapes much of health and aging and reminds us to think about just how much worse things can be for people at the very bottom of the economic structure. As Cottom (2017) notes, economic and social class often become powerful blind spots for researchers seeking to make sense of the world while living and working in middle, upper middle, and upper-class social locations themselves.

In fact, my most powerful lessons about society in graduate school and as a professor have consisted of the constant, continuous, and to my eyes powerfully obvious classism that permeates all aspects of the academy itself. Whether we look to the ritual tradition of hosting academic conferences only in expensive cities or the ways many universities require people to pay up front for such conferences to be reimbursed later, classism shapes how one can or cannot develop an academic career. Likewise, whether we look at the use of school rankings (i.e., who can get into and afford to attend the best schools no matter where they are located) as a proxy for merit on the job market or the requirement for moving—and thus being able to afford to move—to attend programs or take jobs, class dynamics play a powerful role in what it means to even be an academic in contemporary U.S. society. Although I could continue providing examples, one thing I learned fast was that almost all of academic life and career development has at least as much to do with class background as it does with anything one may do in a classroom, for a research project, or that is otherwise considered "academic."

Of course, this just means that academia—as an institution and a setting of work—simply mirrors the rest of U.S. society (Padavic and Reskin 2002; Padavic 1992; Padavic 1991). Although that fact might upset some academics who would like to believe otherwise (i.e., likely folks who grew up middle class or above, went to top ranked schools, and now sit in nice jobs

and live in nice neighborhoods themselves), it is neither surprising nor unexpected. It is, however, an important part of the health and aging process that
impacts everyone in society regardless of occupational or educational credentials (Link and Phelan 1995), and thus an important aspect of understanding my own or any other experience of sex, gender, and sexual health and
aging over the life course (see also Quadagno 2006). In my case, this aspect
of my experience with health and aging plays out in varied ways.

The most obvious way class status and background plays out in my health
and aging can be seen in the example that opened this chapter. Due to my
class status, two things were automatically different for me than for most
academics I have met in my career. First, I was excited to make the low
salary that graduate students make because that was a bigger salary than I
had ever made before. Second, I was almost disallowed to attend graduate
school because I did not have the financial resources to purchase or otherwise possess health insurance. Both of these things shaped my academic
career in ways that diverged from others. In the first case, I was much less
stressed about money than other graduate students who were used to having
more money before graduate school or who passed up on options that would
have paid them more than graduate school. In the second case, I had to take
loans to attend graduate school even though I had department funding and a
national fellowship, which shaped what my income would look like after
graduate school before I even took a single class in the program.

Each of these examples relate to health and aging because they impact
how one experiences financial and other resources over time (Link and Phelan 1995). The requirement to obtain debt to pay for health insurance both
meant that I would have the stress of debt later in life and that I was entering
graduate school without the same benefits of prior health insurance that other
students might have had throughout their lives. At the same time, the interpretation of graduate school funding as a higher salary than I had before
meant I was less stressed about graduate school and finances than some other
graduate students, and that I was coming into the program already managing
more stress from prior economic disadvantage than other students. Especially
considering the powerful role stress plays in overall health and aging (Keith
1993; Pearlin, Menaghan, Lieberman, and Mullan 1981; Ueno 2005), here
we again see contradictions and complicated relationships between my social
locations and my likely health and aging pathways created by external
circumstances.

Class also shaped and continues to shape my interactions and relationships with other people I work with in the academy. In some cases, this is
because I often don't behave and act in ways that are common, ritualized,
and expected in middle and upper class contexts, which may lead to disagree-
ments, confusion, and other issues. This can lead to stress wherein I often
realize after the fact that I did not know the proper forms of speech, dress, or

other ritualized behaviors expected within a given academic context or conversation. As a result, I often feel isolation and worry that impacts my moods and energy long after such encounters because prior training or socialization in upper class norms is not part of the background I bring into work contexts even though it is one of the implicit expectations in such settings.

More importantly in terms of my own health and aging, however, is the fact that I become very angry, and sometimes deeply sad, whenever anyone who has had better economic opportunities than I have complains about difficulties they have in relation to opportunities and resources I was never granted in the first place. In fact, this type of thing can lead me to sad, stressed, and angry emotions even when it occurs with the people I care about the most in my personal life. When someone complains about a difficulty they have because of an opportunity or resources I never got a chance to have, I feel for them and appreciate their need to express such frustration. I know that it is healthy and important for them to share such feelings. At the same time, however, I also feel significant pain because from my class-based perspective or standpoint, they are complaining about being luckier in the class structure than I was, which makes me think about how much different things might have been for me if I could have complained about the luck they have instead of wishing I had it. In these ways, my relationships with others in the academy and the ways I feel, emotionally and physically in such interactions, are impacted by class inequalities over time.

Although I could offer many more examples of the ways class intertwines with other social locations in my own health and aging, here I will provide one final example that spends at least some time in my mind every day—my sex and gender identities. As noted above, I have always experienced my body as female and my own gender as that of a woman. I don't know if I was born this way, as folks say, or if there was some other way this occurred. I just know how I have always felt and seen myself. I wasn't aware that others saw me any other way until I got in trouble a few times as a child for referring to myself the way I preferred. I remember those punishments to this day. I also remember the confusion I felt at the time. I was much older, in my teen years, when I first encountered pamphlets and other materials on transgender experience, and transgender women specifically. I was in my late teens and twenties when I sought to use whatever means possible to live, at least part time, as the woman I saw myself as in a way that would be seen as womanly to others in the United States. I was in my early to mid twenties when my face was injured in an assault, and daily, never-ending, chronic physical pain in that part of my body became a common aspect of my life. For this reason, when I got the chance to attend college and potentially get access to money and other resources that would allow me to feel better, I relocated my womanhood to secrecy and privacy as a way to focus all the energy I had on school, financial survival in school, and a better life some-day.

I think about these experiences because I often wonder about a few differ-ent things as I look back on my life from my current upper-middle class standpoint. Would I have ever gone to college if I could have afforded transition and the necessary medical care to fix my face in my twenties? I don't honestly know, but I think the answer is equally likely to be yes or no. Would I have gone to the schools I went to if finances were not a primary element of my decision-making process? How might my career look differ-ent if I could have afforded to go to the top ranked schools where the people who have most of the highest paid jobs in my field and others get to go to? How long might I have already been living openly—and in a way others could see based on their own ideas of what women look like—as the woman I am if I had some kind of financial security before now? How many of the things that have been bad for my overall health and life expectancy would not have happened if I could have afforded to transition, go to a nice college right out of high school, go to top ranked graduate programs after college, and had health insurance that whole time? Would further transition options still be so scary if I didn't have debts sitting in the back of my mind each time I think about what I want my future to look like?

Each of these questions demonstrate different ways class has shaped the sex, gender, sexual, and health intersections of my life over time. In fact, one could theoretically take each of these questions and form a whole dissertation or longer-term research agenda exploring these questions among other lower, working, and lower-working class sex, gender, and sexual minorities in a wide variety of ways. Although class is often treated simply as a variable in quantitative assessments, it is much less commonly analyzed as a lived expe-rience in relation to health and aging (see Cottom 2017 for a similar point in relation to education). As such, one cannot help but wonder what we might learn about sex, gender, and sexual health if class, as a lived experience intersecting with health and aging, became a more prominent part of such research agendas in the future.

We Also Have to Talk about Race

If we are to take class more seriously as a lived experience in relation to health and aging in the United States as well as in terms of the ways class intersects with sex, gender, and sexual identities and experiences, we can take pointers from important scholarship demonstrating how race shapes every aspect of social life, health, aging, and other social locations in the United States (see, e.g., Grollman 2012; Grollman 2014; Quadagno 1994; Ray, Sewell, Gilbert, and Roberts 2017; Sewell 2017; Sewell and Jefferson 2016; Sewell, Jefferson, and Lee 2016 for reviews). Specifically, researchers convincingly demonstrate that race influences every health outcome, and that people of color—and especially Black people—generally experience more negative health outcomes and disparities in healthcare access than other racial groups no matter what potential mediating factors are taken into account in such analyses (see also Goosby, Cheadle, and Mitchell 2018; Phelan and Link 2015 Williams and Collins 1995).

Such scholarship also highlights the ways that race combines with class, region, sex, gender, sexualities, and other social locations to benefit some at the expense of others. In fact, such studies would suggest that the fact that I generally pass as white (i.e., appear white to other people and am legally assigned white) means that I do not experience class, sexual, or gender disadvantages to the same extent or in the same way as others even though my racial and ethnic background is more complex than my appearance. Rather, the operation of white privilege would lessen the stress I face in relation to class, gender, and sexual health-related marginalization in comparison to other trans, bi, and lower-working class people who do not benefit from the elevated status of whiteness in society (see Schrock et al. 2014; Sumerau and Grollman 2018; Sumerau and Mathers 2019 for discussions of these intersections of gender, sexuality, class, health, *and* race). As Intersectional theorists have repeatedly shown (see, e.g., Crenshaw 1989; Collins 2004; Cottom 2019), race intersects with every other aspect of social identity in ways that impact both the individual effects of each social location and the ways class, sex, gender, sexualities, health, and other social experiences are racialized in their operation.

This means that alongside each of the complexities noted above, and in every case where sex, gender, sexualities, class, and health intersect, we must also examine how such dynamics and contradictions play out differently for people occupying varied racial social locations (see also Grollman 2014; Phelan and Link 2015; Williams and Collins 1995). My case, for example, may offer insights for navigating health and aging as a lower-working class trans woman who passes as white most of the time and is legally white, but it is incomplete without then comparing my experiences to Black trans women and then comparing those experiences to trans women of other races as well (see also Sumerau and Mathers 2019). Although this is one example of the ways the insights above may be extended and more fully utilized, the same can be said about experiences of sexual fluidity, polyamory, different types of health and illness and trauma, and varied manifestations of class disadvantage in varied social settings.

In fact, one reason we situated this chapter in the middle of the book is because this same insight can be applied, as suggested in chapters 1 and 3, in all our case studies. An important next step beyond this book involves asking how race impacts, for example, chronic illness and safe sex practices over the life course (see also chapter 1); intersex status and realization alongside health and aging over time (see also chapter 3); and every other aspect of sex, gender, sexual, and health intersections noted throughout this book. As the first author of this book has noted previously (Nowakowski 2017), health research too often focuses on only one racial population—and does so absent intersecting contexts. Specifically, they have noted how understanding the complexities of health and aging requires attention to ways such processes are shaped and influenced by race as well as other social locations at the same time, at all times, and in relation to all populations and medical conditions.

Rejecting Simplicity

Throughout this chapter, I have sought to demonstrate the importance of rejecting simplicity when thinking about health and aging. Building on the works of many others over time, my goal was to highlight the usefulness of centering attention upon the ways multiple social locations interlock in anything we might call "health" and any process we might name "healthy aging" in a wide variety of ways. Whether we are talking about sex, gender, sexualities, class, race, or any other aspect of our lived experiences, we are talking about facets of our lives that are complex, and that impact our health and aging in complex, nuanced, and sometimes contradictory ways. As such, this chapter is not only a case study of a non-binary, bisexual, and poly trans woman who moved from the lower-working class to the upper middle class and generally passes as white, but also, it is a call for embracing and examining the complexity of health and aging as well as the ways we interpret and define such terms.

To this end, I would ask readers within and beyond academic contexts to consider the multitude of ways sex, gender, and sexualities may influence what constitutes health as well as the ways race, class, and other patterns of social inequality find voice in such meanings. In so doing, we may begin to move beyond static, limited notions of what counts as health, and instead, focus on the multitude of pathways and possibilities for living healthy lives, receiving adequate healthcare and treatments, and responding to health concerns and inequalities in varied communities. Rather than health for some populations and some people who may fit preexisting models, this would represent the development of health research, practices, and systems that might benefit all people in the ways most fitting to their own complicated needs and lives.

Chapter Three

Making Sense of Healthy Embodiment after Realization of Intersex Status

I found out I had intersex traits when I was twenty-four years old. Intersex is a term used to describe a wide range of variations in sex characteristics that do not fit the sex binary categorization of all bodies as only either male or female (InterACT and Lambda Legal 2018). Estimates vary with how many people have intersex traits, but researchers have noted that about 1 out of 150 to 200 people are born with intersex characteristics (Costello 2019; Sumerau and Mathers 2019). Some scholars and advocates claim that people who are born with intersex traits are just as common as people born with red hair or green eyes (Davis 2015). Intersex traits can exist within a person's anatomical features, chromosomes, and/or hormones. These intersex characteristics may be visible during various stages of the life course, such as infancy or puberty, or not at all (InterACT and Lambda Legal 2018).

My intersex characteristics include having what is considered by clinicians to be high levels of testosterone as an AFAB (i.e., assigned female at birth) person and genitals that do not match or conform to what social and medical authorities would consider to be "typical" for a person assigned female or male. In other words, I had and still have a large clitoris for an AFAB individual by most medical and scientific standards. Historically, clinicians and researchers would define this characteristic as "ambiguous genitalia," but intersex advocates have since rejected using this term and find this term to be offensive and pathologizing due to the harmful history of doctors medicalizing intersex bodies and experiences (Intersex Society of North America 2008; see also Karkazis 2008 for historical examples).

Intersex is also a category established in contrast to another term, endosex. Endosex people are people who do not have intersex traits and whose bodies conform to the sex categories that are typically assigned at birth.

Many social institutions and norms are built around endosex people and bodies. Some examples include reproduction (Costello 2014), health and medicine (Davis et al. 2016), families (Costello 2019; Davis and Jimenez 2019), religion (Intersex & Faith 2019), sports (Costello 2010), and public spaces (Sumerau and Mathers 2019). Specifically, these social structures often reinforce binary normative assumptions about which bodies belong in female and male sex categories (Karkazis 2008). Social and medical authorities predominantly enforce and reinforce these ideas or what may be called endonormativity, which refers to the ways endosex people disallow and erase intersex experiences throughout society (Davis 2015). Public health and medicine are both still built around endonormative values and beliefs, which ultimately harm the health and well-being of intersex people. Within the context of healthcare access and operation, medical authorities treat intersex bodies as an abnormality that needs immediate medical attention (Davis et al. 2016).

For example, I am a survivor of unnecessary genital "normalizing" surgery as a result of having intersex traits. This surgical procedure that I, nor my parents, consented to occurred less than a week after I was born. Many intersex infants and adolescents have been subjected to this form of genital mutilation from physicians around the world due to endonormative assumptions of sex and gender in medicine (Costello 2016). However, it is unclear at this time as to how many intersex people have been forced to undergo unnecessary genital surgeries. Often these surgical interventions are disguised by providers as medically necessary and even lifesaving in some cases when discussed with parents or guardians in the process of obtaining consent to perform such "interventions" (see Costello 2019; Davis 2015 for discussion).

Although, historically, clinicians have been encouraged to engage in such unnecessary genital surgeries, much literature in the socio-medical sciences suggest there are no physical benefits to such surgeries (Roen 2008). In fact, many researchers and practitioners describe these medical procedures as harmful and traumatic for intersex people due to various negative physical, reproductive, sexual, and psychological health consequences that emerge as a result of undergoing these medical procedures (Costello 2014; Davis 2015). Further, these consequences are often irreversible and permanent. As such, intersex individuals face significant disparities in health (Davis 2015; Inter-ACT and Lambda Legal 2018) and a lack in affirming healthcare access across the United States (Costello 2019).

Despite the challenges and barriers intersex people often face, visibility and social acceptance has increased for intersex populations in recent years, especially intersex young people. These positive changes in public acceptance of intersex experiences, bodies, and populations are mainly due to the work of intersex advocacy organizations like InterACT: Advocates for Intersex Youth, which aims "to advocate for the human rights of children born with intersex traits" and provide resources for parents, providers, and educators of intersex youth around the globe (InterACT 2019). Intersex populations have been designated as a health disparity population by the U.S. National Institutes of Health (NIH) as of 2016 (U.S. Department of Health and Human Services and National Institute on Minority Health and Health Disparities 2016) and the United Nations has declared unnecessary genital surgeries on intersex youth as a human rights violation (United Nations for LGBT Equality 2017). Awareness and knowledge about the experiences and health of intersex youth and intersex people more broadly continues to grow within and beyond medical education, training, and practice contexts. To date, the majority of research examining intersex populations focuses on the experiences of intersex infants and youth (Davis 2015; Davis and Jiminez 2019).

At the same time, researchers have paid little attention to older adult intersex populations and how intersex people age throughout the life course. Latham and Holmes (2017) suggest that this trend is due to the notion that intersex variations are "problems of childhood, which can be fixed by hormonal and surgical interventions" (84). This observation aligns with most research focusing on intersex young people rather than intersex populations in different stages throughout the life course. Much like transgender; lesbian, bisexual, gay, and queer (LBGQ); and other aging minority populations, older intersex adults have unique health challenges which often require additional medical attention from providers (Latham and Barrett 2015b; Nowakowski et al. 2019; Talley and Casper 2012). Specifically, older intersex populations often live with the consequences of medical violence and trauma due to unnecessary genital surgeries or the withholding of medical documentation over time (Talley and Casper 2012). Despite intersex populations becoming more common in mainstream discourse, older intersex adults often have little to no information about intersex experiences, issues, and needs while rarely being included in medical decision-making processes (Latham and Barrett 2015a).

As a result, research on intersex older adults or intersex aging is almost nonexistent in the socio-medical sciences. This may be due to a combination of factors. Specifically, some older intersex adults are unaware that they have intersex variations due to the long history of intersex erasure, stigma, discrimination, and medicalization (Latham and Barrett 2015a; Latham and Holmes 2018; Talley and Casper 2012). Another reason could be due to older intersex individuals categorizing or reframing their intersex traits as a medical or chronic health condition, such as Disorders of Sex Development or Differences of Sex Development (DSDs). Many intersex people, especially intersex young people, have rejected this terminology while others, especially older intersex people, describe their intersex traits as a medical condition instead of a social characteristic or identity. Specifically, there are people who do treat intersex traits as medical conditions, and thus reject intersex as a sex identity (Davis 2015). Among intersex communities, there still continues to be an ongoing debate about whether intersex should be treated and described as an identity or a chronic health or medical condition.

My self-discovery of intersex traits led me to claim my intersex status as a sex identity. In other words, I am intersex. I am also transgender and non-binary. Some intersex people identify as transgender, others do not. Even though sex and gender are separate and discrete social categories (Sumerau and Mathers 2019; West and Zimmerman 1987), realizing my intersex status as a transgender person was a kind of a relief, but also made me extremely worried and uncertain. On the one hand, the realization of my intersex status confirmed my past decision to not conform to the sex and gender identities that I was assigned to at birth (i.e., endosex female and a cisgender woman). I reject the "born in the wrong body" narrative as an intersex and trans researcher and educator because this rhetoric can be harmful for people who do not fit neatly within the medical model of transgender identity (Johnson 2015). I was also relieved that my body did not conform to bio-essentialist beliefs that have harmed trans and non-binary communities (see Sumerau and Mathers 2019 for further discussion).

On the other hand, this self-discovery opened the floodgates to many questions and uncertainties about my body, health, and future. How can I experience healthy aging as an intersex person? Which providers are intersex and trans-affirming? Do I have a higher risk of reproductive and sexual disparities as an intersex and trans person? Could I have prevented my chronic health conditions from impacting my life if I knew about my intersex status earlier in my life? These questions and uncertainties about my own body made me wonder about how intersex people navigate the realization of their intersex status and how these self-discoveries shape their health and aging over the life course.

As an openly queer, trans, and intersex scholar and a medical sociologist, my prior work focuses on the health, aging, and care experiences of lesbian, gay, bisexual, transgender, queer, intersex, and asexual (LGBTQIA) populations throughout the life course. In this chapter, I reflect upon scholarship concerning healthy embodiment in the context of intersex aging populations. Building on previous works that center older intersex adult populations, I use autoethnographic accounts from my own lived experience about the realization of my intersex status to fill existing gaps in the literature while offering some ways discomfort in one's body, sexual and gender fluidity, and sex/gender incongruency can impact health, aging, and a sense of self.

EXAMINING STANDPOINT

As an intersex and trans person, I recognize my body is seen as a political war zone of sorts, despite intersex and trans populations existing throughout recorded history (Stryker 2008; Costello 2016). Social and medical authorities have forced me to conform to sex and gendered expectations, which I believe aided my own self-destruction and led me to experience many negative health consequences throughout my life. For example, I have been managing, battling, and attempting to recover from an eating disorder throughout the past decade. Although media depictions often suggest that only white, cisgender, heterosexual, middle class, young women struggle with eating disorders, many people with varied social identities experience eating disorders and often do so in a wide variety of ways (Smolak and Striegel-Moore 2001). In my case, surviving bulimia and anorexia in a body that does not conform to endonormative and cisnormative assumptions substantially shaped my lived experience of myself, my identities, my body, and my relationship to food and health.

At the same time, I am also a college campus rape survivor. Specifically, I was raped less than a year after I started my undergraduate career in Florida. That was also my first sexual encounter with another person, although politically I wouldn't count this event as a sexual experience, but more so sexual violence. This traumatic event alongside negative experiences with campus security and university officials dismissing my Title IX case led me to develop forms of Post-Traumatic Stress Disorder (PTSD). Specifically, I often have night terrors where I scream and sweat profusely. Further, vaginal-penetration style sexual intercourse is almost always painful for me. I am thus one of many LGBTQ people who have been subjected to sexual violence at some point in their lives. In addition, many rape survivors develop significant physical, mental, and reproductive/sexual health disparities as a result of sexual violence. My own experiences with such events thus also shaped my understanding about my health and aging over time and in relation to varied embodied experiences.

Like many of my trans and non-binary community members, I have also experienced variations of gender dysphoric feelings over the years. Not having access to gender-affirming binders, binding tape, or clothes, I remember all the times during my childhood, I would duct tape my chest to be flatter and try on my brother's clothes while my parents were at work. I remember spending many hours screaming and crying after cross-country, track, and wrestling meets, because no matter how hard I worked, I wouldn't be able to completely conform with what is considered a manly body according to societal standards. In many ways, these experiences impacted my own relationships with my body, health, and identities in ways that I would not be able to understand or name until years later.

As suggested in each of these examples, health and aging are processes that occur over time and also heavily influence the ways the body and mind shift in relation to new biological, psychological, and social events, knowledges, understandings, and experiences (Nowakowski 2019a). How I view my own health and aging processes has been influenced by my own understandings and experiences of multiple forms of marginalization over the life course. As a perspective, focusing on the life course offers ways for people to move through and make sense of status passages and other life events over time and in relation to existing social norms. For example, I have changed and enhanced my own perspectives about my body and personal biographies over time utilizing information and experience later in life to reflect upon and understand experiences in previous moments. In my scholarship and applied work, I thus focus my efforts on exploring how queer, trans, and intersex people age and view their health throughout the life course. In this chapter, I hope to offer a unique perspective that health researchers and practitioners can utilize to serve intersex aging populations as more people become aware of their and other people's intersex statuses.

For the remainder of this chapter, I thus examine how I learned about and responded to my status as an intersex person. In so doing, I also focus on the ways discomfort in one's body, sexual and gender fluidity, and sex/gender incongruency impact health, aging, and a sense of self. Further, I highlight the ways people may, in healthy and unhealthy ways, respond to situations where they feel that their body does not fit who they are, and where interactions with medical providers focused on said body can become moments of conflict and tension. I organize these reflections in chronological order of my journey finding out and coming to terms with my intersex status and how my lived experience shapes my life course trajectory.

Endonormativity in Social and Medical Settings

Literature in the socio-medical sciences points to the various ways medical interventions impact and often harm intersex infants and youth. Health professionals are often unaware or otherwise know very little about how to care for patients with intersex variations (Davis 2015; InterACT and Lambda Legal 2018). In consequence, medical authorities often attempt to make their intersex patients conform to endosex female/male binary expectations (Costello 2016; Costello 2019). Specifically, medical authorities have engaged in endosexist practices in attempt to make intersex patients appear to have endosex bodies that fit in a normative model of sex (Costello 2019; Davis et al. 2016). Scholars of law and bioethics have written extensively about the harm of medicalizing intersex bodies, identities, and experiences (Davis 2013). Prior literature describes the medical decision-making processes of providers performing unnecessary medical interventions on intersex infants and youth, and highlights the ethical dilemma wherein medical authorities perform unnecessary procedures that have no direct health benefits for intersex people (Costello 2016; Davis et al. 2016). In consequence of endonormative assumptions in public health and medicine, intersex people face significant challenges addressing their health and healthcare needs because clinicians often lie or withhold information about their medical histories and intersex status (Costello 2019; Davis 2015).

I first started to realize that my body did not fit in an endosex female/male binary framework when I was in middle school at a slumber party at a friend's house. During that time, my endosex female friends were very curious about our bodies, and more specifically, our chests and genitals. They wanted to see who looked the most "womanly" and attractive. As silly as this comparison is, young women and girls have a high risk of viewing their bodies in a negative fashion and having a poor body image as a result of unrealistic expectations of what a woman is supposed to look like. At the slumber party, one of my friends happened to bring a handheld mirror with her for the sleepover. Using this mirror, we began inspecting and comparing our genitals while grabbing and squeezing our own chests.

I was the last one to proceed with this inspection. This was because I was a very anxious, self-conscious child at the time. When it was my turn, I pulled down my underwear and held the mirror under my genitals in-between my legs. As soon as my friends got a good look at my genitals, they became mostly silent. However, one of them broke the silence when they gasped, and then said, "Nicole [my legal and chosen first name at the time], what is that?! Your lady parts look strange!" After this person spoke, everyone else roared with laughter and asked to get a closer look. Horrified by the situation, I ran into the closest bathroom, called my mom, and asked her to pick me up from the party. I blamed my departure on not feeling well. At the time, I didn't have the language or knowledge to understand the gendered and sex nuances of what happened during that night or why my genitals did not look like my friends' genitals.

The story above is an example of the ways endonormativity is embedded in social interactions and how it can be harmful for people who do not fit neatly in sex and gender binaries. By engaging in normative assumptions of what bodies, more specifically genitals, should look like, my childhood friends fail to fully account for the fluidity and diversity of people's anatomical features. Further, this instance is a case of endosex people's expectations of binary sex categories and bodies and how normative accountability (Johnson 2015) is enforced through their expression of what they think a (cisgender) woman should be. In fact, this would be an example of what Sumerau and Mathers (2019) call "doing endosex," or the process whereby people enforce endonormative assumptions of sex on themselves and others in social interaction. In this and other cases, by holding intersex populations accountable to a binary medical model of sex identity, endosex people create a situation wherein intersex people often face negative experiences that contribute to poor health outcomes as they age.

In fact, despite growing scholarship in queer, trans, and intersex studies, literature on reproduction, health, and medicine has been slower in examining the broad diversity of sexual, gender, and sex minority populations (Costello 2014; Lampe et al. 2019; Wingo et al. 2018). Further, hierarchical and ideological structures of sex, gender, and sexuality as minority statuses influence individuals' reproductive experiences and health outcomes, especially for those who challenge notions of sex, gender, and sexuality in contemporary society (Costello 2014; Sumerau and Mathers 2019; Wingo et al. 2018). In consequence, LGBTQIA populations experience significantly high risks for poor reproductive health outcomes, and often experience significant challenges when seeking reproductive and other healthcare providers Johnson and Rogers 2019; Wingo et al. 2018).

In the case of intersex reproduction, medical practitioners often assume most intersex people are infertile and are unable to reproduce without medical intervention. However, many intersex individuals are capable of undergoing pregnancy and childbirth without medical assistance (Costello 2014). In addition, current breast cancer and prostate cancer screening guidelines fail to account for bodies other than those found within female and male endosex populations (Costello 2014). The sex, gender, and sexual identities of individuals can thus greatly impact their reproductive health and care from providers in various healthcare environments (Costello 2014; Nowakowski and Sumerau 2018; Nowakowski and Sumerau 2019c).

In my case, when I was in high school, I was the last one out of my women's cross-country team to start visibly menstruating. I was fifteen years old at the time. I remember I was so thrilled at the time because I could finally relate to my friends, and at the time, I equated womanhood and femininity with menstruation. This was at least partly due to the little reproductive and sexual health education I had as someone who grew up in a rural and working-class area with political and religious conservatism embedded into the practices, norms, and rituals of everyday life (see Lampe 2019b for discussion). I was thus unaware that not every AFAB person had to undergo menstruation of some sort after puberty. A couple of months after I started menstruating, my menstruating cycles visibly stopped due to complications from my eating disorder and the impact on my body from running competitively for my high school cross-country and track teams.

Shortly after my visible menstrual cycle stopped, I went to an obstetrician-gynecologist for the first time. After she examined me, she asked if any family members had complications with pregnancy and childbirth. When I said no and asked why, she said not to be surprised if I have trouble staying pregnant or having children when I get older. She also noticed some scar tissue around my clitoris region. Even though I never wanted to give birth or be a parent to a child that I can remember, I was surprised and puzzled by the interaction. When I tried to probe my obstetrician-gynecologist by asking follow-up questions to better understand her comments, she said I didn't need to worry about this minor detail. Then, she apologized for saying anything in the first place. After additional probing throughout the clinical interaction, I finally gave up and assumed any issues I had were due to my eating condition, even though I failed to disclose that information to my provider at the time. I had no other way to make sense of her statements.

This experience is an example of how endonormative assumptions in healthcare and medicine often make it more difficult for intersex patients to receive adequate and affirming care. By not clearly communicating with me what was going on with my body or why she was asking me questions about my family's fertility history, my obstetrician-gynecologist withheld medical information from me that would have allowed me to gain clarity about my medical history and intersex status. In so doing, her actions illustrate attempts medical practitioners may make to maintain endonormative and cisnormative beliefs about how we should view our bodies and sex identities, and in my case, how I viewed these things as someone with anatomy that did not fit into an endosex female/male binary system.

Self-Discovery of Intersex Status

Narratives of intersex people's lived experiences often serve as powerful tools for researchers, educators, and health professionals to adequately study and provide affirming care to intersex populations. As I became more familiar with LGBTQIA experiences, identities, and issues during my undergraduate and graduate programs, I started to realize my experiences and interactions in social and medical settings about my autonomic features were similar to other intersex people I have met in research and advocacy communities. I distinctively remember watching Dr. Georgiann Davis's TED Talk for a course where I was a graduate teaching assistant during my first semester of graduate school at the University of Central Florida. I was captivated by her knowledge and clear explanation of intersex experiences, while sharing her own experiences as an intersex scholar and advocate.

In the video, Dr. Georgiann Davis spoke about how doctors lied to her and removed her testes without her knowledge or consent through an unnecessary medical intervention and how she later learned about her intersex status a few years after that surgery after obtaining her medical records. Dr. Davis then went on to share details from her experiences with finding, researching, and advocating for intersex communities to "bridge [her] personal experience with intersex was [her] professional passion in understanding gender inequalities." Because of her work and along with the work of Dr.

Cary Gabriel Costello, I found the tools and insights that allowed me to understand and connect to other intersex people and communities in my work as an intersex sociologist. For this reason and many others, I am forever grateful for their impactful contributions of intersex studies in sociology and feminist scholarship.

A year later, I interviewed sixty transgender and gender-nonconforming young adults about their healthcare experiences for my grant-funded, master's thesis project. During that time, I interviewed two respondents who also identified as intersex. Both respondents had very similar experiences to my own without me actually knowing whether I had intersex traits at the time, and both had also been subjected to unnecessary medical interventions due to their intersex statuses. My thoughts ran wild during those interviews while I tried to be engaged as much as possible. I was sweating during the first interview because I was nervous about discussing something, that is, intersex identity and experiences, that I wasn't professionally or emotionally prepared for. By the second interview, I kept thinking about starting the process to obtain my medical records and trying to remember which hospital I was born in. When I was memoing about my thoughts and feelings about each of their interviews, I kept thinking and reflecting on the similarities of their experiences with my own.

These events became a catalyst for me to investigate further about whether or not I had intersex traits. By that point, I read countless journal articles about intersex populations and watched hundreds of hours of videos with intersex advocates discussing their experiences, knowledge, and advocacy work. Despite the amount of preparation I put into knowing what to expect when determining whether or not I had intersex traits, nothing would prepare me for the emotions and stress of uncovering my medical history. After speaking to colleagues I trust who frequently train medical students and clinicians about sex and gender diversity, I began my own quest of self-discovery to understand my medical history and body.

As many people in intersex communities have noted previously (Davis 2015), the first step to possibly determine whether someone has intersex, endosex female, or endosex male traits is to obtain your medical records, starting with your birth records. However, it is often extremely difficult to obtain birth records as an intersex person due to existing gatekeeping mechanisms that medical and administrative authorities often put in place. This is despite federal medical privacy laws requiring care facilities to send medical records within forty-five days after a person requests them. Since I was born during a time when hospitals and other medical facilities had hand-written records instead of electronic records, it became more difficult to retrieve my birth records. In addition, administrative staff at the hospital where I was born kept avoiding my emails, phone calls, and letters requesting access to these records. I finally discovered my intersex status and history of surgical trauma as a newborn after repeated attempts to retrieve my birth records over the course of six months.

Around the same time that I started to doubt that I would ever see my birth records, I received an email on March 8, 2019, that my birth records request had been fulfilled. I was in an evaluation team meeting with Xan, the first author of this book, when I saw the email. I told Xan that the email arrived and asked if they would be willing to look over my birth records first so I would have someone to discuss them with when I was ready. Since Xan is a medical research scientist and faculty member at a medical school as well as someone who lives with a chronic health condition (see chapter 1 for more information), they have become very well-versed in reviewing medical documents. As such, I thought they would be the perfect person to help me decipher my birth records into information I could comprehend and use (Lampe 2019a).

With Xan's assistance, I found out, based on the information I gathered from my medical records and from my parents' recollection of what happened, that as a healthy newborn I was in the hospital for five days after I was born. At the time, doctors told my parents that I needed a tympanostomy or more simply put, tubes in my ears. My parents trusted my providers at the time because, like many working and middle-class families, they believed in the ethical and honest reputations of doctors who spent years in medical school. Within my birth records, there was a vague notation of me having "ambiguous genitalia" as a baby, but there was no written evidence to suggest that I had a tympanostomy during that time. In fact, my birth records indicated that my temperature was taken with an ear thermometer. The problem with that is babies generally don't have their temperature taken via their ears if they recently had a tympanostomy, as this might put them higher risk of ear infections. In other words, my doctors lied to my parents, and instead of an issue with my ears, my records suggested that medical providers performed surgery on my genitals without explicit consent to do so (Lampe 2019b).

As Xan explained the news to me, I was horrified, but I was also quite relieved. I was horrified because I had experienced a traumatic medical procedure that I did not consent to as a newborn. I had no idea what effect this might have had on my mental and physical experience of life after that point. I also felt like I didn't even get a chance to not have any reproductive and sexual health complications in my life (see Lampe 2019a for discussion). I also thought of what it would have been like to be assigned-male instead of assigned-female. I wondered how this might have influenced the way I grew up, what I thought of myself and my body, and how I fit within my family and hometown as I aged over time. All these unanswerable questions filled my head at the same time, and I spent much time later considering each one.

It is important to note that a majority of intersex newborns are assigned female at birth by medical authorities (Davis 2015; Costello 2016). In my case, a team of doctors decided my sex and gender identity before I had a chance to be an independent person. When I found out about my intersex traits, I also blamed myself for not knowing this medical information for twenty-four years. Even though I did not believe in sex and gender binary belief systems, I felt relieved because I felt like my gender identity as a genderqueer, transmasculine, non-binary person was slightly affirmed. To my mind, the records said my body had never been meant for binary identities in the first place. Stated another way, I felt like I "passed" in my own head or that now I possessed a more legitimate claim to my transgender identity. The combination of all these feelings created confusion, anger, joy, and other reactions within me that took me much time to decipher and process.

These experiences also reveal some ways endonormativity and cisnormativity operate as systemic processes that are so engrained in our social norms and expectations that we often catch ourselves, regardless of our individual identities, falling into a set of binary normative frameworks. But at the same time, I was mainly relieved that this self-discovery process was mostly over. I always had questions, but now, at least, I had a few answers to go with them. As such, I found some clarity knowing more about my medical information and background. By learning more about my own medical history and existing literature of intersex populations (see also Davis and Jimenez 2019; Topp 2019), I was able to effectively begin to educate providers about my health needs as a patient with an intersex, trans, and queer biography (Lampe 2019b).

INTERSEX AGING

My experience discovering my intersex status and history of medical trauma via genital reconstructive surgeries gave me clarity on what my health and aging care needs are as someone with intersex, trans, and queer biographies. These experiences also raised questions that most providers I know wouldn't be able to answer. What are the experiences of aging intersex people? What kind of care do I need to better my reproductive and sexual health as I age as an intersex person? Do I have any additional reproductive and sexual health condition risks as an intersex person? Would my doctors provide intersex and trans affirming care for me when I am an older adult? What questions about aging as an intersex person have not even crossed my mind yet?

Seeking to build this type of knowledge, Latham and Barrett (2015b) use narrative data from the Intersex Ageing and Aged Care Project, which aims to document the experiences and needs of older intersex people to inform an evidence-based guide to intersex inclusive aged care services. Two interviews were conducted for a study wherein a narrative from an intersex person in their sixties known as Pat was presented for consideration. Pat noted that increasing attention on intersex populations has been centered about intersex and birth, while little is known about the health and quality of life of intersex people as they age. Pat also expressed concern with the possibility of health professionals seeing Pat's body as an intersex person, especially the uncertainty of how providers will see them in a residential aged care facility. Pat acknowledged that health professionals who have seen their body view their anatomic features as a spectacle.

Like Pat, I have experienced providers treating my body as unique or as a spectacle. The issue with these experiences is that providers are supposed to be equipped with an array of body types and patient experiences. Treating patients as an oddity or exoticizing patients reproduces social and health inequalities among minority and underserved populations (see also Costello 2019; Pearce 2018; Sumerau and Mathers 2019). For the longest time, I avoided reproductive healthcare providers because I was embarrassed and fearful due to interactions with past providers. Further, these processes fuel medical violence against intersex populations because if providers continue viewing their intersex patients as special cases or as oddities, then medical authorities will continue to poorly care for intersex patients and continue genital corrective surgeries among intersex infants and youth. There is a critical need for intersex-specific medical education and services, especially for older intersex populations.

Stated another way, if medical and social authorities continue to treat intersex bodies as medical problems, then these normative assumptions of assigned-sex will erase the experiences of intersex adults and those who experience medical trauma via unnecessary medical genital surgeries. Such consequences will continue to reproduce existing health and aging inequalities among intersex populations, while barring the need for intersex-specific health services for intersex adults as they age. At the same time, the questions I pose above will simply remain unanswered mysteries for each of us who age as intersex people in a society that attempts to ignore our existence within and beyond medical contexts. These issues thus demonstrate a serious area of need for medical science and practice in the coming years.

Transformations in the Life Course

Since I discovered I have intersex traits, I continue to navigate young adulthood with a newfound understanding of myself as an intersex, bi+, and trans person and patient. Specifically, my intersex identity has paved the way toward understanding my lived experiences of managing an eating disorder and dysphoric feelings while surviving a college campus rape. Eating disorders, for example, often are heavily influenced by societal expectations of beauty and social identities. It made sense that I often felt I was too small to be a man, but also did not fit the ideal version of womanhood and femininity. By understanding my intersex history and identity, I began unraveling all the endosexist and cissexist expectations that were placed on me throughout my young adulthood, while understanding how I internalized these expectations in the process.

For example, all my awkward interactions with other assigned-female people started to make sense. Regarding my gender dysphoria, being assigned a sex identity that my body didn't fit contributed to me grappling with attempts to conform to and later reject cisgender expectations of womanhood and manhood. I experience dysphoric feelings substantially less often since self-discovering my intersex identity. Instead of disconnecting my feelings and gender identity from my body and autonomical features, I adapt my body and appearance based on how I am feeling and what I want my gender expression to be. Half of my closet is masculine clothing and the other half is more feminine. When I do experience dysphoric feelings, I develop coping and accountability mechanisms, so I won't spiral into negative mental health domains.

Finally, my intersex status complicates the narrative of my sexual assault. Campus security, for example, originally blamed me for trusting a person and for inviting him into my dorm when all my roommates were out of town for the weekend. They interrogated me for four hours the day after the rape and asked what I was wearing, how many drinks I had, and continued to victim blame me in the process. I can still hear the things they said. "Surely a good looking, young woman like yourself gets a lot of dates?" "How tight was your dress?" "Why didn't you scream?" "Surely someone would have noticed what happened." "Do you have a boyfriend?" "Are you sexually active?" When I was trying to fight off my rapist in my dorm bedroom, he ripped down my gray sweatpants and pulled down his soccer shorts, while pinning me on my bed with my stomach facing the ceiling. Once he glanced down at my genitals, he violently flipped me over. I assume now he did this so he wouldn't see what my childhood friends saw (enlarged clitoris with scar tissue surrounding it) while he was raping me. My rapist then proceeded to violently rape me from behind where he could just ignore my genitals. When I discovered that I have intersex traits, it became clear that societal trends in sexual violence operate through sex and gender binary expectations.

This horrific event is just one case of how normative expectations of sex, gender, and sexualities can manifest in sexual and gender violence for people whose bodies do not neatly fit in binary categories. Whether I think about the gendered nature of the questioning I encountered from campus safety officers or the violent actions of the rapist, I am reminded that my lack of fit within existing sex, gender, and sexual narratives became relevant in negative ways throughout the experiences of sexual assault. Especially as many sex, gender, and sexual minorities experience varied forms of sexual violence in the course of their lives, these dynamics again pose questions about aging—and aging after traumatic events—within such communities. As I've noted throughout this chapter, such questions will need answers if we are to create and provide adequate healthcare for all people regardless of sex, gender, and sexuality.

Aging Between and Beyond Binaries

My lived experiences shaped my understanding of what it means to age between and beyond binaries as someone who experiences sustained liminality or a frequent disruption in a status passage trajectory created by no existing social or medical script for sex, gender, and sexual non-binary aging (see also Barbee and Schrock 2019; Sumerau 2020 for discussion). There is no script that I can abide by in a clinical setting as someone who is intersex and non-binary. Likewise, experiences for someone like me are almost nonexistent in aging studies. More older adults are starting to openly identify as intersex and/or sexual or gender non-binary in social and medical spaces. Even so, I must continue to navigate aging as one without a fixed, binary script for probable health and life status passages to come.

This is because sex and gender binaries leave no room for fluidity as healthcare is structured around static rituals throughout the life course. Instead of these long-standing rituals, providers must try to learn from the experiences of intersex, trans, and queer older adults. For patients who experience intersectional marginalization as they age, interactions with providers are political acts. Providers who are not equipped to care for different minority and underserved populations must make room for patients to teach them. Further, providers must learn to listen to these patients in order to learn about their health and aging journeys. Medical students and faculty I have interacted with since my self-discovery, for example, are often eager to listen to my experiences as an openly intersex, trans, and queer young person. These interactions and my involvement with InterACT Youth give me hope for the future of medicine for intersex people while at the same time showing me just how much work there is to do in these fields.

Concluding Thoughts

How does self-discovery of intersex identity shape my views on aging and life-course trajectories? Discovering my intersex identity and history of surgical trauma as a non-binary person shaped my current understandings of health, body dysphoria, and aging as an eating disorder and rape survivor. Specifically, my lived experiences and the limited literature that exists to date demonstrate the nuances of sex identity in health and aging processes and how intersex people often experience many barriers and challenges navigating medical and social authorities from clinical visits to traumatic events to existing in public spaces. I still wonder what my health needs will be as I age as an intersex person and whether I will find clinicians who are knowledgeable about the experiences and bodies of intersex populations or will at least listen and attempt to learn about such experiences and bodies.

During a time when more people and institutions are paying attention to intersex and trans people, but still attempting to regulate our bodies, there is still an uncertainty of what intersex aging experiences and life-course trajectories might look like. Studying trans, non-binary, and intersex populations may thus expand understandings of health and aging scholarship. For example, I often hear conversations from older queer and trans Southerners at the LGBT center I volunteer at concerning uncertainty of what healthy aging and basic wellness should look like for them, given the limited resources and scarcity of competent, queer, trans, and/or intersex affirming providers in the Deep South.

Whether we are talking about stories of legally unmarried life partners dying and their children or other authorities making their burial arrangements or inheriting all of their belongings, or situations where past healthcare experiences have created enough fear for people to avoid providers at all cost, we are talking about the difficulties of aging while queer, trans, and/or intersex in the United States. The same is true for instances of gender non-conforming couples being separated at hospitals when one of them is ill and for trans people unable to find providers who even know what transition can entail. Each of these examples and many others create very real fears throughout our communities. These fears remain relevant and apparent for LGBTQIA people and families even as many things have improved for our communities over time. By deconstructing social and medical scripts of sex, gender, and sexuality, we can thus begin to better provide impactful and sustainable care to intersex, trans, and queer youth and adults as they age in varied ways and throughout the passage of time.

Conclusions

There are some things you cannot foresee when you embark upon a long-term research project. A global pandemic is one of those things. And yet, as we began to do the final polishing and revisions on this book, a global pandemic took hold of the world, and in so doing, foisted discussions about health, aging, wellness, illness, and disparities in each of these areas to the center stage of most people's minds (Pirtle 2020). With this in mind, we turned our attention to the existing manuscript pages while many people work from home in hopes of lessening the impact of the coronavirus and many other people occupying lower paid and more precarious jobs—like the ones our second author survived on before graduate school (see chapter 2)—suddenly became more visibly "essential" to the economy, well-being, and other aspects of life.

As we accomplish the revisions and rewrites of this final chapter, we are each working from home, keeping our distance from other humans, and adjusting to all the changes and concerns raised by the global pandemic. At the same time, researchers have already begun documenting how societal factors like race (Yancy 2020), class (Hopman et al. 2020), sex (Bali et al. 2020), gender (Wenham et al. 2020), and sexualities (Bali et al. 2020) create disparities in the impact of the pandemic upon different social groups (Pangborn and Rea 2020; Rouleau Whitworth et al. 2020; Sewell 2020). Even as these reports emerge, social media combined with contacts from rural and working class communities both the second (i.e., in the Southeastern United States) and third (i.e., in the Midwestern United States) authors left behind as their careers developed show us significant losses of life, employment, financial options, and other necessities throughout our nation. Everywhere we look, the global pandemic highlights, as we have throughout this book, the need for dramatic transformations in the way U.S. society conceptualizes and accomplishes health.

Our own lives, for example, illustrate major transformations—whether temporary or longer term—that have already occurred in relation to this health crisis. The first author of this book, for example, continues to work to help others acquire healthcare, conduct evaluations and other research related to healthcare access and experience, and advocate for people with cystic fibrosis and other chronic health conditions. At the same time, they do this from home now, reliant upon technology and other resources to both accomplish their work and maintain social distancing for their own and others' health. As they compose manuscripts and videos for educational consumption and advocacy, they thus also manage both their own condition—per usual and in relation to potential risks tied to the pandemic—and their own isolation as one of many people who have shifted from traditional workplaces to remote work.

In fact, their own chronic health condition, in some ways, smooths their experience of shifting to online and socially distanced work overall. This is because people with cystic fibrosis generally cannot be in the same shared space, and as a result, this population of people generally hold meetings, social occasions, support groups, and other functions online and socially distanced from one another at all times. As a result, the first author has adjusted to being online and remote throughout their personal and professional endeavors, but at the same time, this has been a smooth transition because much of their work and social engagement (i.e., the elements with other people with cystic fibrosis) was already done this way before the pandemic. As a result, much of society is, in a very real way, getting a taste of some of the dynamics of social life for people with cystic fibrosis at present, which may allow them to more critically consider the elements of interaction and social life they take for granted at other times even as other populations experience a different social world at all times.

At the same time, the second author of this book navigates a similar shift from traditional workplaces and engagement to online and remote efforts as a professor at a private teaching university. This has meant that the second author of this book and her colleagues—many of whom never did online teaching of any kind before now—shifted their entire pedagogical, educational, emotional support, and interactional models of face-to-face, applied and personal based, and immersive skills based instruction to online models with little time or warning preceding such adjustment. Among other things, this transformation has necessitated the second author, and many other teachers throughout the world, to spend considerable time and energy helping students manage emotional and mental health related to the pandemic specifically while also continuing our usual teaching and support endeavors and doing all this without the ability to meet in person with such students in the process.

At the same time, the third author of this book reflects the experiences of many graduate students at present. While the economy, interpersonal norms, and other aspects of daily life collapsed around all of us, they were in the process of completing required courses for their doctoral studies. This necessitated making certain that all software and other requirements they might have normally been able to acquire or troubleshoot at the university were available to them from their own home. This also meant that, like many graduate students, they found themselves in a place where they know very few people, and where their family and other loved ones are far away. As such, the third author faces the global pandemic, the ongoing requirements of their doctoral study, and their own efforts to maintain health and well-being alongside considerable isolation and growing uncertainty about what academic and other job markets might look like following these recent events. In all such cases, the third author navigates ongoing transformations of health and social life coupled with ongoing occupational demands.

Although we could provide many more examples of the impact of the pandemic upon ourselves and others occupying various social positions, our point here is the same one we have made throughout this book—the existing systems of health in the United States require significant transformations in order to meet the needs of the entire population. The same way we utilized detailed autoethnographic case studies to illustrate sex, gender, and sexual health inequalities embedded in the current system, the pandemic illustrates just how widespread such sex, gender, and sexual inequalities, alongside inequalities tied to class, race and nation (see also Cogburn 2019; French et al. 2020; Powell et al. 2019), are throughout the United States and across a wide variety of social and demographic differences. We thus utilize this final chapter to draw out insights from the discussions in the prior chapters, but also to emphasize again the importance of transforming health systems, practices, and expectations in relation to the differential and unequal social locations, positions, and resources of different groups.

To this end, we next turn to a discussion of insights from the autoethnographic case studies contained in chapters 1, 2, and 3. In so doing, we highlight how the experiences captured in this book draw attention to broader patterns in need of examination and intervention throughout the U.S. healthcare system. Then, we build on these insights to suggest future studies that could begin to illuminate such dynamics throughout society while also suggesting potential interventions for use. Finally, we close this book with a brief discussion about the importance and difficulty of transformation in health and other social systems in hopes of encouraging others to consider the possibilities that exist beyond our current sex, gender, and sexual health norms, and the potential of healthcare systems that work for all.

THREE CASES, SOCIETAL INSIGHTS

In the preceding chapters, we provided three specific case studies concerning the negotiation and experience of sex, gender, and sexual health in the United States. Whether we focus on how people with chronic conditions navigate sexual activity in safe and healthy ways, or how recognition of intersex and other bodily experiences can shift perceptions about sex, gender, sexual, health, and other aspects of life, these chapters provide insight into aspects of health situated betwixt and between existing medical norms, assumptions, and models (see also Sumerau and Mathers 2019). Likewise, when we talk about how class shapes sex, gender, and sexual health or how chronic conditions or traumatic events create similar and different impacts on such experience, these chapters demonstrate the importance of holistic thinking in terms of what constitutes health and the practice of health and medicine in relation to diverse populations (see also Nowakowski and Sumerau 2017b). As such, the cases in the chapters of this book provide entry points for expanding studies and approaches to sex, gender, and sexual health over time and in relation to different social groups.

If, for example, we think about the broader implications of the first case study (see chapter 1), we may begin to ask important questions about what constitutes sexual activity, safe sex, and healthy sexual bodies. Especially as the first author of this book outlines how complex each of these things are in their own life as a sexually active person navigating a chronic health condition, we may ask how similar or differently people managing other chronic health conditions may experience, negotiate, or otherwise manage such complexity. At the same time, the recognition that even things some might find gross can be sources of intimacy, sexual arousal, and bonding for others suggests there may be much to learn about how people think about and treat their bodies in relation to existing notions of health, aesthetic appearance, cleanliness, sickness and well-being, and even bodily diversity (see also Gill 2015). In these and other ways, the first author's discussion of living as both sexual and ill at the same time reveal unanswered questions that might have wide ranging implications for others in society.

We can see similar widespread implications in the second author's elaboration of the ways race, class, sex, gender, and sexual experience all blend together to complicate what does and does not count as healthy at any given time (see chapter 2). Especially as the pandemic itself reminds all of us just how much race and class impact all aspects of health, what might systematic studies of racial, classed, sexed, gendered, and/or sexual *experience* (i.e., the life beyond the numbers in surveys) tell us about the current operations and limitations of existing healthcare systems and norms (see also Nowakowski and Sumerau 2019a). Likewise, how might class status and background—as well as access to resources more broadly—influence what is or is not healthy for anyone at any time and in any given social, geographic, or other setting (see also McMillan Cottom 2017). As noted in chapter 2, a given case can simultaneously represent behaviors that would deem them healthy, unhealthy, or somewhere in between. How might this recognition of the fluidity of what health means impact how we, as a society, approach and understand potential public health policies and proposals? Right now, there is no answer to this question, but a healthcare system that works for all would need to have such answers in order to mitigate the varieties of experience between different groups.

Such complexity becomes even more important when we think of populations—like intersex people—that have historically been labeled as unhealthy regardless of anything they might do as individual people or groups of people (see chapter 3; see also historical and contemporary examples related to racial minorities [Washington 2006] and sexual minorities [Halkitis 2013] and cisgender women [Samuels 2014]). In such cases, we again find a situation where we currently possess no model for health or healthy aging over time. Rather, members of such populations must navigate their own paths, and as suggested in chapter 3, it is imperative to learn from them what these paths look like and adjust healthcare norms to create space for such people within societal definitions of care and health. To this end, however, we will have to, as noted in all three case studies, address the myriad ways that trauma—of various types—can impact physical, social, mental, and other aspects of health and aging. Once again, however, doing so requires expanding healthcare and medical norms, assumptions, and practices to reach the spaces between and beyond any one or two types of "normal."

In all these examples, the case studies in this book reveal potential pathways to developing and bettering health systems for all members of society. Rather than singular examples, they are cases that reveal important questions in need of study and intervention throughout our existing medical and otherwise health-related models. It is with this in mind that we turn to future studies in the next section. Specifically, we outline some ways researchers could begin answering the questions illustrated by these cases in their research endeavors. In so doing, we suggest future studies may seek to go beyond existing models in search of missing pieces within and potential transformations for U.S. medical and health practices.

Looking toward the Future

As researchers who have collectively published over 100 works in social, physical, and medical sciences to date, here we seek to suggest research projects and questions that could allow for the transformation of knowledge concerning sex, gender, and sexual health over time. It is our hope that such efforts could then feed the ongoing cycles of intervention and policy implementation that facilitate, maintain, and/or change existing operations in health systems. In fact, we would suggest that much of the importance of research of any kind may be found in the way such knowledge becomes translated into a concrete, practical actions in the broader world (Crenshaw 1989; Leavy 2015; Nowakowski and Sumerau 2017a). With this in mind, we use this section to highlight a few pathways for future study that could both broaden our understanding of sex, gender, and sexual health and provide the foundation for individual and collective medical and other health-related interventions.

As such, we begin by repeating calls for more empirical survey designs that the first and second author have made at previous points (see, e.g., Nowakowski et al. 2016; Sumerau et al. 2017). Put simply, each of the authors of this book represent populations that would not exist in most of the survey data collected in social, physical, and health sciences to date. This means that it is incredibly difficult to gain any quantitative insight into the health and other experiences of most intersex, transgender, and otherwise sex, sexual, or gender diverse people. This also means that our existing surveys are skewed via their limitation to only parts of the sex, gender, and sexual spectrums operating in society (Westbrook and Saperstein 2015). Stated another way, we cannot assess how accurate they might be for an empirical world of sex, gender, and sexual diversity because they are usually limited to an imaginary world where only portions of such populations exist (Sumerau and Mathers 2019). We thus again call for systematic transformation of quantitative data collection to incorporate the sex, gender, and sexual diversity of our actual, empirical world in hopes that in so doing, we may gain a picture—rather than a limited guess—of what sex, gender, and sexual health looks like across society and quantitatively in relation to other social demographic factors.

Alongside such adjustments to quantitative sampling, we see a wide variety of ways qualitative researchers may continue to expand the purviews of mainstream scientific assumptions and norms through targeted study of sex, gender, sexual, and health diversity. Researchers could, for example, develop content collections of medical and other commentary on sex, gender, sexual, and health variation to examine how such meanings shift, change, and otherwise develop over time (see also Halkitis 2013; Roen 2008; Washington 2006 for examples). Researchers could also utilize the plethora of information in news media, social media, film, television, and other locations to develop composite explorations of how sex, gender, and sexual health finds voice and gets delivered to the broader public at any given time (Leavy 2015). In fact, these and other types of historical and contemporary content analysis may be especially important in demonstrating both the way meanings and assumptions change over time, and the importance of once again transforming normative messages about these topics in society (Foucault 1978; Samuels 2014; Warner 1999).

Especially as sex, gender, and sexual diversity remains lacking in most quantitative surveys and assessments, we also see an important need for interview studies on a wide variety of topics related to health and diversity. How do doctors make sense of sex, gender, and sexuality? How do notions of sex, gender, and sexualities become embedded in existing medical education, protocols, and norms (see also Almeling 2011)? How do intersex people experience interactions with doctors over the life course? How do transgender people of different gender identities? How do sexual minorities? How do doctors make sense of sexual health, and what do they say when greeted by the realities of same-sex sexual activity, sexual activity related to intersex and transgender bodies, and/or sexual activity among people with chronic illnesses? When we think of medical providers, what do they know about sex, gender, and sexual health? When we think of people seeking medical provision, how do their sex, gender, and sexual lives complicate or ease such endeavors? The reality is that each of these, and so many more, questions could become the basis for a full dissertation or book-length interview-based research studies in the social and medical sciences.

Although it would take considerably more interactions with sex, gender, and sexual minorities than survey methods often require (Kleinman 2007), we see such interview studies as especially important both to supplement surveys lacking sex, gender, and sexual diversity, and to gain rich, nuanced portraits of the experience of sex, gender, and sexual health over time. When we look at the current pandemic, for example, the second author automatically thinks about how she has put off some aspects of transition related healthcare unexpectedly, and how common this experience is among trans people navigating the pandemic around the world right now. What might in-depth interviews with trans people in this circumstance tell us about healthcare access, trans health, and the impact of a health crisis upon other sectors of the healthcare system? How might trans people narrate and make sense of these experiences? These are only two questions, but they share a point—in-depth interviews allow researchers to gain insight into the experiences beyond the numbers for people navigating any type of healthcare interaction.

In a similar vein, the complexities in the cases throughout this book, as well as the examples above, suggest there is an important role for ethnographic and autoethnographic studies of the variety of health experiences in society (see also Jenkins 2018). Whether we are seeking to understand how sex, gender, and sexuality become relevant in medical settings or how medical practitioners respond to sex, gender, and sexual health issues, ethnographic and autoethnographic works can provide a view of what happens on the ground in concrete situations. Whether we seek to understand how people manage and intertwine their sex, gender, and sexual health in relation to their biographical and social standpoints or how sex, gender, and sexual health factors influence interpersonal interactions, such studies can show us what goes on in the unusual and usual spaces that make up a life. Finally, as we have done in this book, such efforts can be utilized to demonstrate areas in need of study throughout society.

Of course, the combination of these factors and the cases presented here also demonstrate the importance of narratives for understanding and studying sex, gender, sexual, health, and other social phenomena. As the global pandemic hit, for example, it was not surprising that many scholars we know turned to Jessica Smart Gullion's sociological novel *October Birds* for inspiration, guidance, and understanding. This novel, focused on the way pandemics emerge and play out over time in relation to socio-cultural factors, represented an available social science based narrative other people could draw from, build upon, and otherwise utilize to study and understand what we were facing. Although this is only one example, history is riddled with the power of narratives to mobilize action, provide insight to mass audiences in times of uncertainty, and leverage pursuits of transformation and change within a given society and related to specific norms (see also Leavy 2015). Narratives thus provide insights into the operation of the world, but also opportunities to reimagine and reframe those operations for the betterment of ourselves and others (Adam 2011).

As we have done throughout this book, we would thus empathize the importance of continuing to collect, disseminate, and support diverse sex, gender, sexual, and health narratives that may be useful in imagining better healthcare systems in the future. Whether such works are fictional, autobiographical, interview-based, memoirs, ethnographic, autoethnographic, or media based, each type of narrative—and as many different perspectives as we can collect along lines of race, class, and region—may shed light on elements of problems occurring more broadly and insights capable of helping us reimagine who we are and how we do things in relation to sex, gender, and sexual health as a society. As we have noted throughout this book, sex, gender, sexual, and health narratives provide a powerful tool for understanding what we do now, and for imagining what we could do better in the future.

Concluding Thoughts

Throughout this book, we have examined and discussed the importance of transforming sex, gender, and sexual health. In so doing, we have drawn on our own experiences as people navigating these factors, and as scholars studying such topics over time. The combination of these endeavors reveal many missing elements in existing medical and otherwise health-related knowledge in the social, physical, and medical sciences, but they also demonstrate how greater incorporation of the experiences of sex, gender, sexual, and health diverse populations may begin to fill these gaps and provide possibilities for better healthcare systems. As such, our work here joins the chorus of voices calling for a reformation of the ways we do health as well as sex, gender, and sexual research, practice, and provision in the United States.

Especially in the face of a global pandemic impacting all elements of the social world, these insights both become even more clear and join rising recognition, throughout society, of the limitations of current U.S. healthcare systems, assumptions, and norms. As we each sit in our own homes, barred from our former lives and normal places of work, we recognize that transformation has come to the world of health and social life whether or not any given person advocated or desired such change beforehand. At the same time, we recognize that even in such a historical moment, the transformations that we need for a healthcare system and systems of health and medicine that would benefit all are even larger. To this end, here we have sought to outline some aspects of U.S. healthcare in need of transformation, and we end this volume with hope that such endeavors, no matter how difficult, may occur over time.

Methodological Appendix

As suggested in the opening vignette at the beginning of this book, the seeds for this project were planted via a series of conversations between the three authors and other intersex, trans, and queer people in Florida throughout 2017 and 2018. At the time, the first two authors were working on narrative and community projects concerning healthcare access while also aiding their own students and others in search of sex, gender, and sexual affirming healthcare and health-related information. Likewise, the third author was starting graduate studies and engaging with LGBTQIA community groups with a focus on the healthcare experiences and options for transgender youth in the Southeastern United States. and in Florida specifically. The combination of these efforts led to a series of conversations about the topic, the relative absence of scholarly materials on these topics, and ideas about how to engage with these two realities as scholars, community members, and teachers.

As part of these conversations, we began to learn many details about both the care options available to people of diverse sex, gender, and sexual identities. At the same time, the third author began working for and with the first author at Florida State University College of Medicine on projects related to community healthcare access, evaluation, and provision. During a series of conversations at the office, between work on other projects, the first and third author began to outline notes for a potential book-length project on the healthcare experiences and needs of people occupying differential sex, gender, and sexual social locations within society. With this roughly formulated idea in hand, the first and third author approached the second author as, at first, a sounding board for ideas for the book, and later, a collaborator and co-author for a book emphasizing the complexity of sex, gender, sexual, and health intersections in the course of people's broader social, political, and emotional lives.

At the time, Xan (the first author) was becoming more and more active in cystic fibrosis communities while working on both promotion for the upcoming release of their first novel, *Other People's Oysters* (co-written with the second author, 2018), autoethnographic analyses of their experiences with Cystic Fibrosis, and a new collection of health-themed poetry. They were also crafting multiple academic articles narrating the intersections of chronic illness, healthcare experience, and sex, gender, and sexual experience in relation to health. Drawing on the combination of these experiences and efforts, they proposed a book where we utilized our own "unconventional" (in terms of academic and scholarship norms) social locations as case studies for calling other researchers to more critically examine intersections of sex, gender, sexualities, and health in society. To this end, they suggested a collaborative project wherein we constructed, co-revised, and collectively situated our own health experiences as a mechanism for furthering socio-medical understanding of sex, gender, sexual, and health diversity.

At the same time, J (the second author) was in the process of creating, revising, and beginning to prepare do promotion for three forthcoming (at the time) books examining sex, gender, and sexual diversity in society (see, e.g., Sumerau 2018; Simula, Miller, and Sumerau 2019; Sumerau and Mathers 2019). In each of these projects, J had worked with colleagues to emphasize the diversity of sex, gender, and sexual narratives available in contemporary society while situating these works in relation to systemic patterns of social inequality over time. In so doing, J had become well versed in the editorial and compositional dynamics of book length projects integrating narrative and scholarly techniques to illuminate specific populations and social issues in a given society. Utilizing these experiences, J worked with the second and third authors to outline a plan that would become the contents of this book and to serve as the manager or editor for the collaborative composition of this project.

As these organizational details were taking shape, Nik (the third author) was completing their first stage of graduate study by interviewing a wide variety of trans youth about health, healthcare experiences, and healthcare needs. At the same time, as noted in chapter 3, they were beginning to gather information about their own health history, intersex status, and medical records. They were also working on their first scholarly narrative analysis utilizing sociological concepts to make sense of familial and sexual life (see Lampe 2019b) and their first creative writing about sex, gender, and sexualities (see Lampe 2019a). As a result, they sought to utilize this project to both (1) integrate their creative and scholarly approaches to narrative writing, and (2) utilize the editorial and publishing experience of the first and second authors as a ready source of mentorship for the process of constructing and publishing books.

The combination of each of these individual skill sets, experiences, and dynamics allowed us to create a collaborative approach throughout the formation of this book. Specifically, we intentionally worked to each be involved in all aspects of the construction of this volume from the earliest planning to the final revision processes. In so doing, the first two authors were able to utilize their experience to help the third author effectively learn about a creative process that was new to them. At the same time, the third author was able to be a source of support and critical reading for the purposes of establishing a narrative composition that would be accessible to readers and researchers at various stages of their development. Although these are only examples of the process, they illustrate the overall approach to the work—we worked individually and together to craft a unified narrative wherein our similar and different sex, gender, sexual, and health experiences could reveal areas in need of study.

With this in mind, two processes started at the same time. First, each of the three authors began crafting their own, individual, discussion of sex, gender, and sexual health. In this way, each author focused specifically on their own experiences and the ways they could narrate such experiences while integrating them into a scholarly framework. Second, J began the process of outlining an introduction and conclusion that could speak to the overall themes in the individual narratives, but did so via a loose outline—built from the early notes of each individual chapter—so that the overall composition could be adjusted to fit the evolving contents of the autoethnographic chapters. Especially since we each worked in these areas already, this process allowed us to each focus on our existing strengths and knowledge sources before later synthesizing all these resources for the book itself.

Via the combination of these efforts, we initiated a process wherein we wrote, revised, shared, further revised, and shared again as the autoethnographic chapters took shape. Although we elaborate on this process below, we share the entirety of this origin story here for the purposes of other scholars seeking to do similar work, and because recent methodological scholarship has called for transparent discussions of the entirety of events that go into the construction of social scientific studies (Leavy 2015). Below, we outline the processes utilized for this book for the same two purposes, and in so doing, outline the establishment of this study's data and the manner whereby we created, analyzed, and composed this book from the combinations of such work over the past few years. Before moving to the study itself, however, we share our own standpoints as humans, researchers, activists, and authors seeking to understand and theorize about contemporary social relations in the United States.

Authors' Standpoints

Because all scholarship is rooted in personal values and beliefs whether or not the researchers express their own social locations (Kleinman 2007), we provide subjective statements concerning our identities and some of our values. We do this here because our identities and values shaped the autoethnographic experiences shared in this book as well as many decisions made throughout the work (Collins 2000; Compton, Meadow, and Schilt 2018; Leavy 2014; Moore 2010).

Xan (the first author) was raised in a liberal, secular home just outside the city of New Brunswick, New Jersey, area after spending the first years of their life in the Jackson, Mississippi, metro area. They were their parents' only child, finally conceived through artificial insemination from an anonymous donor as part of a research study after their parents had spent a long time wanting to have a child. Their racial and ethnic background are thus complicated in a variety of ways. Because they universally pass as some variety of white, they describe themselves as a multiethnic white person. Growing up in the Northeast exposed Xan to both the privileges and stigmas associated with being "ethnic white" especially because of their father's uniformly Polish heritage.

Xan spent most of their childhood either at school—first a Montessori school that emphasized independent learning, then a prep school that focused on community service—or at the medical school where their parents taught. They helped out in their parents' neuroscience lab and also participated in a variety of activities for medical students. This gave them a unique perspective on their own chronic disease and the challenges they faced in getting accurate diagnosis and appropriate care. Home was a community with plenty of racial, ethnic, cultural, and religious diversity where most families would be considered upper middle class. Xan's upbringing and values were thus influenced by exposure to different religions, spiritualities, and philosophies as well as the various liberal Catholic traditions present in their own family. Their own lifelong agnosticism reflects this socialization via awareness that multiple truths can coexist.

Xan was assigned female at birth and still thinks this is an accurate description of their sex. However, like their parents, they never developed much of a gender identity concept. They continue to identify as agender as they did in childhood, but are more open about it these days and can better describe what it means for them. Because their parents always made it very clear that being attracted to people of the same sex or gender was acceptable and welcome, they also felt little anxiety in the gradual process of figuring out that they were bisexual. Over the years, Xan's parents have supported them in relationships with people of different sexes and genders (as well as races, ethnicities, cultures, etc.) and in having more than one partner at a time.

Likewise, their parents taught them about trans experience at an early age. They provided some basic explanations of how sex, gender, and sexuality may exist in different combinations for different people. This helped Xan understand that even though all of their partners had what looked or felt like a penis at the time they were first together, that did not mean they themselves were straight. Rather, their partners over the years have had a range of gender characteristics and sex identities alike, as well as sexualities. Over the years, Xan's parents have also enjoyed learning more about the nuances of these attributes from J (whom Xan has been with since 2011 and married in 2016) as they have gotten to know her better.

J (the second author) was raised in a conservative, Southern Baptist home in rural South Carolina after she was given up for adoption in her first years of life. She realized early in life that she was not like other people when it came to gender and sexuality, as she was attracted to both cisgender men and women; and, when she met some later in her youth, J found herself attracted to intersex and transgender people, as well. J was assigned male at birth (AMAB), but never identified as such in any personal way. In her late teens, she almost transitioned to a female, but also became familiar with non-binary gender identities around that time and eventually adopted such an identity for varied reasons and for just over a decade. In recent years, however, she has continued to move toward transition in various ways and will continue this process in the years to come. Today, J identifies as a non-binary transgender woman, and a bisexual person (on the pansexual end of the bi spectrum).

J is married to the first author (see above for the first author's standpoint discussion). J and her spouse share a committed life and relationship, though they are also polyamorous and maintain romantic-sexual relationships with others at present, as well. J also openly identifies as an agnostic, and she is legally and visibly (most of the time) seen as white, though her ethnic and racial background is more complicated in other ways. Finally, J was raised in the lower-working-class but has moved up in the class structure throughout the past decade of her life and currently would be considered upper-middle-class by most measures of socioeconomic status utilized in the social sciences.

Nik (the third author) was raised in a conservative, upper-working-class, Catholic home in rural, northeast Indiana. Although they were assigned female at birth by medical providers, they learned in their twenties that they possessed intersex characteristics. As a result, many of the times where they felt out of place vis-à-vis sex segregated norms (i.e., in athletics and religious rituals) made more sense, but as a child, they simply felt frustration and tension with others' expectations about their supposed sex and gender. Nik left Indiana after high school to attend college in Tampa on a scholarship, and in so doing, began to move away from their religious upbringing and into an open expression of their bisexuality in college. At present, Nik identifies as spiritual but not religious, and further identifies as a white, middle class, polyamorous, bisexual, intersex, and as a non-binary transgender person.

Following college, Nik moved to Orlando to pursue a master's degree in sociology and a career studying health and aging among sex, gender, and sexual minority populations in society. While in Orlando, Nik began more openly identifying and presenting as a non-binary transgender person, completed a master's degree and thesis on the healthcare experiences of transgender youth, and began working with Xan (the first author) at Florida State University College of Medicine. Seeking to further their educational and professional goals, Nik currently lives in South Carolina where they are pursuing doctoral study in sociology, health, aging, and queer and transgender studies. As we complete this book, Nik works with health and LGBTQIA organizations across South Carolina and Florida while preparing for their doctoral examinations in medical sociology.

Although we differ in many ways, each of the authors of this book also share a few important characteristics. As noted above, for example, each of us experiences the social world as people who are typically identified—structurally and interpersonally—as white, as members of the broader transgender, bisexual and queer, and polyamorous populations, and as people working primarily in academic settings. We are also each survivors of various types of trauma, and people who have each experienced violence and abuse within and beyond relationship contexts at different times in our lives. As such, both the similarities and differences in our standpoints influence both the way we experience intersections of sex, gender, sexualities, and health as well as how we are able to narrate such dynamics in this book.

The Study

With the background or origin story of the study and the standpoints of the authors of this work in mind, we now turn to our discussion of the study itself. As noted throughout this book, the study here focused on how sex, gender, sexual, and health transformations impact social life and often reflect existing social inequalities within and beyond medical settings. We conducted three separate, but related, autoethnographic analyses of how these dynamics play out in each of our own lives, and then utilized these analyses to deliver a unified discussion of the topic throughout the book. In the sections that follow, we offer more depth and discussion of this process, which may be useful to other scholars seeking to do similar projects.

Autoethnographic Composition

As noted above and in parts of the book (see the introduction, for example), this study began with the creation of three separate, yet related, autoethnographic examinations of sex, gender, sexual, and health intersections over time. As is common in autoethnographic traditions (see Adams 2011; Leavy 2014; Nowakowski and Sumerau 2019a), this involved critically evaluating both (1) our own personal experiences, feelings, and reflections, and (2) the location of these events in relation to existing cultures, norms, and expectations. Stated another way, we focused on the way our own biographies could shed light on broader cultural patterns in society (Ellis and Rawicki 2013). In so doing, we sought to capture pieces of ourselves that contain important insights and questions situated within the social world beyond our individual selves.

The autoethnographic work in this book emerged in an iterative process that contained four stages of activity. First, each author worked in isolation drawing from journals (personal and those kept for other studies) and memories to reflect upon and write about their experiences at the intersection of health, sex, gender, and sexualities. In these early drafts, we each sought to develop thick descriptions and initial analyses of such experiences for the purposes of illuminating what it feels like to experience health and social identities at the same time and over time (Adams 2011). These early drafts thus did the work of drawing the ideas from the biographical and scholarly world and bringing them to life in the form of a narrative (Leavy 2015). Although each of these first versions of chapters 1 through 3 took varying amounts of writing and rewriting (i.e., drafts), the completion of a draft we felt comfortable having edited by the team represented the conclusion of stage one.

Second, we subjected our own autoethnographic drafts to the editorial eyes of other members of the team. Referred to commonly as "collaborative autoethnography" (Chang et al. 2013; Cragun and Sumerau 2017; Ellis and Rawicki 2013), this process involved each author sending their draft first to the second author (J) who has worked extensively in journalism, qualitative methodology, and creative writing and editing throughout the past decade (see www.jsumerau.com for examples). J then edited and made comments on each of the autoethnographies (including her own) concerning (1) any confusion in the text, (2) elements of similarity and difference between the three works, and (3) places where more or less scholarly or creative exposition might be necessary. After this process, J sent each of the autoethnographies to the first and third authors who undertook a similar revision process. At the conclusion of this stage, we each had a draft that contained editorial commentary and suggestions from each of the other authors and in relation to the broader contents of the book itself.

Third, each author took the edited version of their initial draft (with all commentary available), and together we discussed the edits and suggestions as a team. As these discussions took place, J also took notes on the themes and contents developing for use in the construction of the introduction and conclusion portions of the manuscript. At this point, the composition process became a negotiation wherein each author and each commenter discussed, debated, and considered all possible methods for completing the autoethnographic chapter in question. In this way, we were able to collaboratively revise and shape the contents and themes throughout the works to both (1) maintain the difference and insight of each analyses, and (2) synthesize the analyses to illustrate broader themes throughout the volume (Chang et al. 2013).

Fourth and finally, each of the autoethnographic analyses was re-written and revised as many times as necessary to establish the final, polished versions shared in this book. In this way, the first three stages were repeated as need be as the form and content of the analyses each took shape over time. As is common in multiple forms of qualitative research (Leavy 2014), we thus engaged in a back and forth process wherein the initial drafts were edited, revised, edited again, and revised again over time to polish, accentuate, and illustrate important themes, connections to existing literature, and the maintenance of a clear narrative voice throughout. In so doing, the contents of the autoethnographic analyses evolved in an organic, inductive processes of reading, writing, revision, and communication over the course of a year.

Bookending the Autoethnographies

Although it has become more and more common to see collaborative autoethnographies—and ethnographies—in shorter forms like journal articles and book chapters over time (Nowakowski and Sumerau 2019a), it remains rare to see collections of such collaborative work in book form. As Leavy (2015) notes, an important part of book length analyses, both creative and purely scholarly in composition, involves the development of an overall narrative capable of advancing existing theory and research, delivering a concise argument illustrated by the contents, and situating the cases used within social and political contexts (see also Kleinman 2007). As a result, the creation of the three autoethnographies chronicled above necessitated the establishment of synthesis chapters (or bookends) framing the overall conversation occurring throughout the book and the broader literature.

For this endeavor, we agreed as a team that J would take the lead on this effort because the bulk of her work—scholarly, literary, and educational—involves synthesizing and translating multiple disciplines, arguments, and other components for different audiences (see, for recent examples, Simula,

Sumerau, and Miller 2019; Sumerau 2019; Sumerau and Mathers 2019). To this end, J maintained an ongoing and evolving set of notes throughout the composition, editorial, negotiation, and revision processes of the autoethnographies, which she turned to at various points of the process to analyze the similarities and differences in these works. In so doing, J compared and contrasted the autoethnographic chapters over time, and observed how each of the three focused heavily on transformations needed or created in the intersections of sex, gender, sexualities, and health over time and in relation to social norms.

With this common theme identified in the finished autoethnographic sections, J wrote preliminary drafts of both the introduction and conclusion to this book. These drafts were then shared with each of the other authors, which allowed them to revise, edit, and suggest adjustments to both these chapters and the autoethnographic texts. We then continued to revise all content chapters in the book in a back and forth manner while each contributing literature—in varied fields—related to the overall theme of transformation in the case of sex, gender, and sexual health, healthcare systems, and societal inequalities over time. We continued this process while also receiving feedback from others—from talks and review of the materials—over time until we arrived at the final version of the book.

A Note on the Pandemic

As noted in the conclusion, an unexpected aspect of the composition of this book arose when the global pandemic developed over the course of the winter and spring of 2020. At the time, we were approaching the final delivery date for the completed, revised, and polished version of the book, and at the same time, the publishing company and each of our universities shifted to remote operation, social distancing protocols, and other combinations of stalled or adjusted processes. As a result, we decided to do two things that were not initially part of this project, and could not have been planned for in the operation of this project before the pandemic struck the world. First, we decided, as evidenced in the conclusion, to briefly discuss how the pandemic itself relates to the study in this book. Second, we followed the early release of scholarship related to the pandemic in order to provide some of this information in the final version of this book before completing its delivery for production.

We did these two things for a multitude of reasons, but the most important ones should be noted here. First, we recognize that many of the transformations we call for and discuss throughout this book have only become clearer in light of the pandemic. Second, because of the shift to remote work and other adjustments, we were granted extra time for the polishing and full delivery of the book than what we had planned for in the first place. We sought to use this time in hopes that doing so would make this volume even more useful during and after the pandemic plays out in the world. Third and finally, as noted in the conclusion, we were all too aware with how the pandemic impacts our own lives, and thus sought, as so many are doing at present, to situate such experiences in relation to our ongoing work in relation to healthcare in the United States.

We thus offer this volume as both a project focused on health transformations that was created, refined, and mostly completed prior to the pandemic, and a project focused on health transformations that are clearer to many people during the pandemic. It is thus our hope that this volume will serve as a useful resource as we all, within and beyond health scholarship and advocacy sectors, now wrestle with the importance of improving and otherwise transforming our existing healthcare systems. We further continue to hope for the best for everyone managing this pandemic throughout the world as we continue to do our parts as researchers active within and around many healthcare sectors, discussions, and organizational structures.

Bibliography

Adams, Tony E. 2011. *Narrating the Closet: An Autoethnography of Same-Sex Attraction*. Los Angeles, CA: Left Coast Press.

Almeling, Rene. 2011. *Sex Cells: The Medical Market for Eggs and Sperm*. Berkeley, CA: University of California Press.

Ashley, Florence. 2019a. "Gatekeeping hormone replacement therapy for transgender patients is dehumanizing." *Journal of Medical Ethics* 45: 480–482.

Ashley, Florence. 2019b. "Homophobia, Conversion Therapy, and Care Models for Trans Youth: Defending the Gender-Affirmative Approach." *Journal of LGBT Youth* doi: 10.1080/19361653.2019.1665610.

Bali, Sulzhan, Roopa Dhatt, Arush Lal, Amina Jama, Kim Van Daalen, and Devi Sridhar. 2020. "Off the Back Burner: Diverse and Gender-Inclusive Decision-Making for COVID-19 Response and Recovery." *BMJ Global Health* 5(5): e002595.

Barbee, Harry and Douglas Schrock. 2019. "Un/gendering Social Selves: How Nonbinary People Navigate and Experience a Binarily Gendered World." *Sociological Forum* 34(3): 572–593.

Barringer, M. N., J. E. Sumerau, and David Gay. 2017. "Examining Differences in Identity Disclosure Between Monosexuals and Bisexuals." *Sociological Spectrum* 37(5): 319–333.

Bird, Chloe E. 1999. "Gender, Household Labor, and Psychological Distress: The Impact of the Amount and Division of Housework." *Journal of Health and Social Behavior* 40: 32–45.

Calasanti, Toni M. and Kathleen F. Slevin 2001. *Gender, Social Inequalities, and Aging*. Walnut Creek, CA: AltaMira Press.

Chang, Heewon, Faith Wambura Ngunjiri, and Kathy-Ann C. Hernandez. 2013. *Collaborative Autoethnography*. Los Angeles, CA: Left Coast Press.

Charmaz, Kathy C. 2006. *Constructing Grounded Theory: A Practical Guide Through Qualitative Analysis*. Thousand Oaks, CA: Sage.

Cogburn, Courtney D. 2019. "Culture, Race, and Health: Implications for Racial Inequalities and Population Health." *Milbank Quarterly* 97(3): 736–761.

Collins, Patricia Hill. 2000. *Black Feminist Thought: Knowledge, Consciousness, and the Politics of Empowerment*. New York, NY: Routledge.

Collins, Patricia Hill. 2004. *Black Sexual Politics: African Americans, Gender, and the New Racism*. New York, NY: Routledge.

Compton, D'Lane, Tey Meadow, and Kristen Schilt. 2018. *Other, Please Specify: Queer Methods in Sociology*. Oakland, CA: University of California Press.

Costello, Cary Gabriel. 2010. "Caster Semenya: Una Perspectiva Intersex." Pp. 69–72 in *Cuerpos Distintos: Ocho Años de Activismo Transfeminista en Ecuador*, edited by Almeida Ana and Vásquez Elizabeth. Manthra Editores.

Costello, Cary Gabriel. 2014. "Not a "Medical Miracle": Intersex Reproduction and the Medical Enforcement of Binary Sex and Gender." Pp. 63–79 in *Queering Motherhood: Narrative and Theoretical Perspectives*, edited by Margaret F. Gibson. Branson, MO: Demeter Press.

Costello, Cary Gabriel. 2016. "Trans and Intersex Children: Forced Sex Changes, Chemical Castration, and Self-Determination." Pp. 109–113 in *Women Health & Healthcare: Readings on Social Structural & Systemic Issues*, edited by Elizabeth Cabell Hawkinson Gathman. Dubuque, IA: Kendall Hunt Publishing Co.

Costello, Cary Gabriel. 2019. "Understanding Intersex Relationship Issues." Pp. 231–245 in *Expanding the Rainbow: Exploring the Relationships of Bi, Pan, Queer, Ace, Intersex, Trans, Poly, and Kink People*, edited by Brandy Simula, Andrea Miller, and J. E. Sumerau. Boston, MA: Brill/Sense.

Cottom, Tressie McMillan. 2017. *Lower Ed: The Troubling Rise of For Profit Colleges in the New Economy*. New York: The New Press.

Cottom, Tressie McMillan. 2019. *Thick*. New York: The New Press.

Courtenay, Will H. 2000. "Engendering Health: A Social Constructionist Examination of Men's Health Beliefs and Behaviors." *Psychology of Men & Masculinity* 1(1): 4–15.

Cragun, Ryan T. and J. E. Sumerau. 2017. "Losing Manhood like a Man: A Collaborative Autoethnographic Examination of Masculinities and the Experience of a Vasectomy." *Men and Masculinities* 20(1): 98–116.

Crawley, Sara L. 2012. "Autoethnography as Feminist Self-Interview" Pp. 143–160 in *The SAGE Handbook of Interview Research: The Complexity of the Craft, 2nd edition*, edited by Jaber F. Gubrium, James A. Holstein, Amir B. Marvasti, and Karyn D. McKinney. Los Angeles, CA: Sage.

Crenshaw, Kimberle. 1989. "Demarginalizing the Intersection of Race and Sex: A Black Feminist Critique of Antidiscrimination Doctrine, Feminist Theory and Antiracist Politics." *University of Chicago Legal Forum*. Available at: https://chicagounbound.uchicago.edu/uclf/vol1989/iss1/8.

Cunningham, Darcy. 2018. "Darcy's Blog: Gunnar is Gross." *Gunnar Esiason Blog*. Retrieved Feb. 21, 2020 (http://www.gunnaresiason.com/darcys-blog-gunnar-gross/).

Davis, Georgiann. 2013. "The Social Costs of Preempting Intersex Traits." *The American Journal of Bioethics* 13(10): 51–53.

Davis, Georgiann. 2015. *Contesting Intersex: The Dubious Diagnosis*. New York, NY: New York University Press.

Davis, Georgiann. 2016. "This Girl Has Balls." TEDxUNLV. Retrieved at https://www.youtube.com/watch?v=RtjVqsIME2A

Davis, Georgiann and Jonathan Jimenez. 2019. "Not Going to the Chapel? Intersex Youth and an Exploration of Marriage Desires and Expectations." Pp. 247–264 in *Expanding the Rainbow: Exploring the Relationships of Bi, Pan, Queer, Ace, Intersex, Trans, Poly, and Kink People*, edited by Brandy Simula, Andrea Miller, and J. E. Sumerau. Boston, MA: Brill/Sense.

Davis, Georgiann, Dewey, Jodie M., and Murphy, Erin L. 2016. "Giving Sex: Deconstructing Intersex and Trans Medicalization Practices." *Gender & Society* 30(3): 490–514.

Dick, Kirby, S. Rose, D. Dorn, and K. Dick. 1998. *Sick: The Life and Death of Bob Flanagan, Supermasochist*. United States: Kirby Dick Productions.

Didion, Joan. 2005. *The Year of Magical Thinking*. New York, NY: Knopf Doubleday Publishing Group.

Ellis, Carolyn and Jerry Rawicki. 2013. "Collaborative Witnessing of Survival During the Holocaust: An Exemplar of Relational Autoethnography." *Qualitative Inquiry* 19(5): 366–80.

Elliott, Sinikka. 2012. *Not My Kid: What Parents Believe about the Sex Lives of Their Teenagers*. New York, NY: New York University Press.

Fields, Jessica. 2008. *Risky Lessons: Sex Education and Social Inequality*. New Brunswick, NJ: Rutgers University Press.

Foucault, Michel. 1978. *The History of Sexuality Volume I: An Introduction*. New York, NY: Pantheon Books.

French, Bryana H., Jioni A. Lewis, Della V. Mosley, Hector Y. Adames, Nayeli Y. Chavez Duenas, Grace A. Chen, and Helen A. Neville. 2020. "Toward a Psychological Framework of Radical Healing in Communities of Color." *The Counseling Psychologist* 48(1): 14–46.

Gates, Henry Louis, Jr. 2013. *Life upon These Shores: Looking at African American History, 1513–2008*. New York, NY: Alfred A. Knopf.

Geertz, Clifford. 1973. *The Interpretation of Cultures*. New York, NY: Basic Books.

Geist-Martin, Patricia, Lisa Gates, Liesbeth Wiering, Erika Kirby, Renee Houston, Anne Lilly, and Juan Moreno. 2010. "Exemplifying Collaborative Autoethnographic Practice Via Shared Stories of Mothering." *Journal of Research Practice* 6(1): Article M8.

Gill, Michael. 2015. *Already Doing It: Intellectual Disability and Sexual Agency*. Minneapolis, MN: University of Minnesota Press.

Goffman, Erving. 1959. *The Presentation of Self in Everyday Life*. New York, NY: Doubleday.

Goffman, Erving. 1963. *Stigma: Notes on the Management of a Spoiled Identity*. New York, NY: Simon & Schuster, Inc.

Goffman, Erving. 1977. "The Arrangement Between the Sexes." *Theory and Society* 4(3): 301–331.

Goosby, Bridget J., Jacob E. Cheadle, and Colter Mitchell. 2018. "Stress-Related Biosocial Mechanisms of Discrimination and African American Health Inequities." *Annual Review of Sociology* 44(1): 319–340.

Grollman, Eric Anthony. 2012. "Multiple Forms of Perceived Discrimination and Health among Adolescents and Young Adults." *Journal of Health and Social Behavior* 53(2): 199–214.

Grollman, Eric Anthony. 2014. "Multiple Disadvantaged Statuses and Health: The Role of Multiple Dimensions of Discrimination." *Journal of Health and Social Behavior* 55(1): 3–19.

Gullion, Jessica Smartt. 2014. *October Birds: A Novel about Pandemic Influenza, Infection Control and First Responders*. Rotterdam, The Netherlands: Sense Publishers.

Halkitis, Perry. 2013. *The Aids Generation: Stories of Survival and Resilience*. New York, NY: Oxford University Press.

Harder, Brittany M., and J. E. Sumerau. 2019. "Understanding Gender as a Fundamental Cause of Health: Simultaneous Linear Relationships between Gender, Mental Health, and Physical Health Over Time." *Sociological Spectrum* 38(6): 387–405.

Heath, Melanie. 2012. *One Marriage Under God: The Campaign to Promote Marriage in America*. New York, NY: New York University Press.

Hill, Terrence D. and Belinda L. Needham. 2013. "Rethinking Gender and Mental Health: A Critical Analysis of Three Propositions." *Social Science & Medicine* 92: 83–91.

Hopman, Joost, Benedetta Allegranzi, and Shaheen Mehtar. 2020. "Managing COVID-19 in Low-And Middle-Income Countries." *JAMA* 323(16): 1549–1550.

InterACT: Advocates for Intersex Youth. 2019. "InterACT Mission Statement and Organizational History." Retrieved Feb. 22, 2020 (https://interactadvocates.org/about-us/mission-history/).

InterACT and Lambda Legal. 2018. "Providing Ethical and Compassionate Health Care to Intersex Patients." Retrieved on Feb 22, 2020 (https://www.lambdalegal.org/sites/default/files/publications/downloads/resource_20180731_hospital-policies-intersex.pdf).

Intersex & Faith. 2019. "Stories of Intersex and Faith." Retrieved Feb. 22, 2020 (https://storiesofintersexandfaith.com/).

Intersex Society of North America 2008. "Is Intersex the Same as Ambiguous Genitalia?" Retrieved Feb. 22, 2020 (https://isna.org/faq/ambiguous/).

Jenkins, Tania M. 2018. "Dual Autonomies, Divergent Approaches: How Stratification in Medical Education Shapes Approaches to Patient Care." *Journal of Health and Social Behavior* 59(2): 268–282.

Johnson, Austin H. 2015. "Normative Accountability: How the Medical Model Influences Transgender Identities and Experiences." *Sociology Compass* 9(9): 803–813.

Johnson, Austin H. and Baker A. Rogers. 2019. "'We're the Normal Ones Here': Community Involvement, Peer Support, and Transgender Mental Health." *Sociological Inquiry* DOI: https://doi.org/10.1111/soin.12347.

Johnson, Austin H., Ivy Hill, Jasmine Beach-Ferrara, Baker A. Rogers, and Andrew Bradford. 2019. "Common Barriers to Healthcare for Transgender People in the U.S. Southeast." *International Journal of Transgender Health* 21(1): 70–78

Karkazis, Katrina. 2008. *Fixing Sex: Intersex, Medical Authority, and Lived Experience, 1st Edition.* Durham, NC: Duke University Press Books.

Keith, Verna M. 1993. "Gender, Financial Strain, and Psychological Distress among Older Adults." *Research on Aging* 15: 123–147.

Kleinman, Sherryl. 2007. *Feminist Fieldwork Analysis.* Thousand Oaks, CA: Sage.

Lampe, Nik. 2019a. "Intersex." *HEAL: Humanism Evolving Through Arts and Literature* 11(2): 13.

Lampe, Nik. 2019b. "You cared before you knew: Navigating Bi+ familial relationships." Pp. 35–46 in *Expanding the Rainbow: Exploring the relationships of Bi+, Polyamorous, Kinky, Ace, Intersex, and Trans people*, edited by Brandy L. Simula, J.E. Sumerau, and Andrea Miller. Boston, MA: Brill.

Lampe, Nik M., Shannon K. Carter, and J. E. Sumerau. 2019. "Continuity and Change in Gender Frames: The Case of Transgender Reproduction." *Gender & Society.* 33(6): 865–887.

Latham, J. R. and Catherine Barrett. 2015a. "Appropriate Bodies and Other Damn Lies: Intersex Ageing and Aged Care." *Australasian Journal on Ageing* 34: 19–20.

Latham, J. R. and Catherine Barrett. 2015b. "'As We Age': An Evidence-Based Guide to Intersex Inclusive Aged Care Services. Melbourne: La Trobe University.

Latham, J. R. and M. Morgan Holmes. 2018. "Intersex Ageing and (Sexual) Rights." Pp. 84–96 in *Addressing the Sexual Rights of Older People Theory, Policy and Practice*, edited by Catherine Barrett and Sharron Hinchliff. London, UK: Routledge.

Leavy, Patricia. 2014. *The Oxford Handbook of Qualitative Research.* New York, NY: Oxford University Press.

Leavy, Patricia. 2015. *Method Meets Art: Arts-Based Research Practice, 2nd Edition.* New York, NY: Guilford Press.

Link, Bruce G. and Jo C. Phelan. 1995. "Social Conditions as Fundamental Causes of Disease." *Journal of Health and Social Behavior* 35(Extra Issue): 80–94.

Lipman, Andy. 2019. *The CF Warrior Project.* Alpharetta, GA: BookLogix.

Martin, Patricia Yancey. 2005. *Rape Work: Victims, Gender & Emotions in Organization & Community Context.* New York, NY: Routledge.

McMillan Cottom, Tressie. 2017. *Lower Ed: The Troubling Rise of For-Profits.* New York, NY: The New Press.

McMillan Cottom, Tressie. 2019. *THICK: And Other Essays.* New York, NY: The New Press.

Miller, Lisa R. and Eric Anthony Grollman. 2015. "The Social Costs of Gender Nonconformity for Transgender Adults: Implications for Discrimination and Health." *Sociological Forum* 30(3): 809–31.

Moore, Mignon R. 2010. "Articulating a Politics of (Multiple) Identities: LGBT Sexuality and Inclusion in Black Community Life." *Du Bois Review: Social Science Research on Race* 7(2): 315–34.

Needham, Belinda and Terrence Hill. 2010. "Do Gender Differences in Mental Health Contribute to Gender Differences in Physical Health?" *Social Science & Medicine* 71: 1472–1479.

Nowakowski, Alexandra C. H. 2016a. "Hope Is a Four-Letter Word: Riding the Emotional Rollercoaster of Illness Management." *Sociology of Health and Illness* 38(6): 899–915.

Nowakowski, Alexandra C. H. 2016b. "You Poor Thing: A Retrospective Autoethnography of Visible Chronic Illness as a Symbolic Vanishing Act." *The Qualitative Report* 219: 1615–1635.

Nowakowski, Alexandra C. H. 2017. "Death Check: Doing Life and Research with Chronic Autoimmune Disease." Pp. 3–14 in *Negotiating the Emotional Challenges of Conducting Deeply Personal Research in Health*, edited by Alexandra C. H. Nowakowski and J. E. Sumerau. Boca Raton, FL: Routledge.

Nowakowski, Alexandra C. H. 2018a. "Original Parts: Aging and Reckoning with Cystic Fibrosis Related Kidney Disease." *Patient Experience Journal* 5(1): 7–10.

Nowakowski, Alexandra C. H. 2018b. "Cystic Fibrosis Kidney Disease: 10 Tips for Clinicians." *Frontiers in Medicine—Nephrology* 5242: 1–3.

Nowakowski, Alexandra C.H. 2019a. "Neverland: A Critical Autoethnography of Aging with Cystic Fibrosis." *The Qualitative Report* 24(6): 1338–1360.

Nowakowski, Alexandra C. H. 2019b. "The Salt without the Girl: Negotiating Embodied Identity as an Agender Person with Cystic Fibrosis." *Social Sciences* 8(3): 78. DOI: 10.3390/socsci8030078.

Nowakowski, Alexandra C. H. and J. Edward Sumerau. 2015. "Swell Foundations: Fundamental Social Causes and Chronic Inflammation." *Sociological Spectrum* 35(2): 161–178.

Nowakowski, Alexandra C. H. and J. E. Sumerau. 2017a. "Out of the Shadow: Partners Managing Illness Together." *Sociology Compass* 11(5): e12466.

Nowakowski, Alexandra C. H. and J. E. Sumerau. 2017b. "Aging Partners Managing Chronic Illness Together: Introducing the Content Collection." *Gerontology and Geriatric Medicine* DOI: 10.1177/2333721417737679.

Nowakowski, Alexandra C. H. and J. E. Sumerau. 2018. *Other People's Oysters*. Boston, MA: Brill.

Nowakowski, Alexandra C. H. and J. E. Sumerau. 2019a. "Reframing Health and Illness: A Collaborative Autoethnography on the Experience of Health and Illness Transformations in the Life Course." *Sociology of Health and Illness* 41(4): 723–739.

Nowakowski, Alexandra C. H. and J. E. Sumerau. 2019b. "Gender, Arthritis, and Feelings of Sexual Obligation in Older Adults." Pp. 177–204 in *Women and Inequality in the 21ˢᵗ Century*, edited by Brittany C. Slatton and Carla D. Brailey. Boca Raton, FL: Routledge.

Nowakowski, Alexandra C. H. and J. E. Sumerau. 2019c. "Older Women's Sexual Health: Gaps and Possibilities." *Women's Health* 15: 1–7.

Nowakowski, Alexandra C. H., Katelyn Y. Graves, and J. E. Sumerau. 2016. "Mediation Analysis of Relationships between Chronic Inflammation and Quality of Life in Older Adults." *Health and Quality of Life Outcomes* 14: 46.

Nowakowski, Alexandra C. H., J. E. Sumerau, and Lain A. B. Mathers. 2016. "None of the Above: Strategies for Inclusive Teaching with "Representative" Data." *Teaching Sociology* 44(2): 96–105.

Nowakowski, Alexandra C. H., Alan Y. Chan, Jordan Forrest Miller, and J. E. Sumerau. 2019. "Illness Management in Older Lesbian, Gay, Bisexual, and Transgender Couples: A Review." *Gerontology and Geriatric Medicine* DOI:10.1177/2333721418822865.

O'Neil, Adrienne, Victor Sojo, Bianca Fileborn, Anna J. Scovelle, and Allison Milner. 2018. "The #MeToo Movement: An Opportunity in Public Health?" *The Lancet* 391(10140):2587–2589.

Orne, Jason and James Gall. 2019. "Converting, Monitoring, and Policing PrEP Citizenship: Biosexual Citizenship and the PrEP Surveillance Machine." *Surveillance & Society* 17(5): 641–661.

Padavic, Irene. 1991. "The Re-Creation of Gender in a Male Workplace." *Symbolic Interaction* 14(3): 279–294.

Padavic, Irene. 1992. "White-Collar Work Values and Women's Interest in Blue-Collar Jobs." *Gender & Society* 6(2): 215–230.

Padavic, Irene and Barbara Reskin. 2002. *Women and Men at Work, Second edition*. Thousand Oaks, CA: Pine Forge Press.

Pangborn, Nicole A. and Christopher M. Rea. 2020. "Race, Gender, and New Essential Workers during COVID-19." *Contexts*.

Pettigrew, Ian. 2012. *Salty Girls*. Access via: https://www.ianpettigrew.com/projects.html.

Pearce, Ruth. 2018. *Understanding Trans Health: Discourse, Power and Possibility*. Bristol, UK: Bristol University Press.

Pearlin, Leonard I., Elizabeth G. Menaghan, Morton A. Lieberman, and Joseph T. Mullan. 1981. "The Stress Process." *Journal of Health and Social Behavior* 22(4): 337–356.

Phelan, Jo C. and Bruce G. Link. 2015. "Is Racism a Fundamental Cause of Inequalities in Health?" *Annual Review of Sociology* 41(1): 311–330.

Pirtle, Whitney N. Laster. 2020. "Racial Capitalism: A Fundamental Cause of Novel Coronavirus (COVID-19) Pandemic Inequities in the United States." *Health Education & Behavior* published online ahead of print, DOI: 10.1177/1090198120922942.

Powell, Wizdom, Jennifer Richmond, Dinushika Mohottige, Irene Yen, Allison Joslyn, and Giselle Corbie-Smith. 2019. "Medical Mistrust, Racism, and Delays in Preventive Health Screening among African-American Men." *Behavioral Medicine* 45(2): 102–117.

Quadagno, Jill. 1994. *The Color of Welfare: How Racism Undermined the War on Poverty.* New York, NY: Oxford University Press.

Quadagno, Jill. 2006. *One Nation, Uninsured: Why the US has No National Health Insurance.* New York, NY: Oxford University Press.

Ray, Rashawn, A. A. Sewell, Keon L. Gilbert, and Jennifer Roberts. 2017. "Missed Opportunity: Leveraging Mobile Technology to Reduce Racial Health Disparities." *Journal of Health Politics, Policy, and Law* 42(5): 901–924.

Read, Jen'nan Ghazal and Bridget K. Gorman. 2010. "Gender and Health Inequality." *Annual Review of Sociology* 36(1): 371–386.

Ridgeway, Cecilia L. 2011. *Framed by Gender: How Gender Inequality Persists in the Modern World.* New York, NY: Oxford University Press.

Rier, David. 2000. "The Missing Voice of the Critically Ill: A Medical Sociologist's First Person Account." *Sociology of Health & Illness* 22(1): 68–93.

Ritter, Lacey J. and Alexandra C. H. Nowakowski. Forthcoming 2021, Under Contract. *Sexual Deviance in Health and Aging.* Latham, MA: Lexington Books.

Roen, Katrina. 2008. "'But We Have to Do Something': Surgical 'Correction' of Atypical Genitalia." *Body & Society* 14(1): 47–66.

Roen, Katrina and Peter Hegarty. 2018. "Shaping Parents, Shaping Penises: How Medical Teams Frame Parents' Decisions in Response to Hypospadias." *British Journal of Health Psychology* 23: 967–981.

Rouleau Whitworth, Tanya, Katherine Cyr, and Anthony Paik. 2020. "Remotely Coping: How Are Students Faring During the COVID-19 Pandemic?" *Contexts.*

Samuels, Ellen. 2014. *Fantasies of Identification: Disability, Gender, Race.* New York, NY: New York University Press.

Sanders, Emile, Tamar Antin, Geoffrey Hunt, and Malisa Young. 2019. "Is Smoking Queer? Implications of California Tobacco Denormalization Strategies for Queer Current and Former Smokers." *Deviant Behavior* DOI: 10.1080/01639625.2019.1572095.

Santos, Theodore C., Emily S. Mann, and Carla A. Pfeffer. 2019. "Are University Health Services Meeting the Needs of Transgender College Students? A Qualitative Assessment of a Public University." *Journal of American College Health* DOI: 10.1080/07448481.2019.1652181.

Schrock, Douglas, J. E. Sumerau, and Koji Ueno. 2014. "Sexualities." Pp. 627–656 in *Handbook of the Social Psychology of Inequality*, edited by Jane D. McLeod, Edward J. Lawler, and Michael Schwalbe. New York, NY: Springer.

Serano, Julia. 2007. *Whipping Girl: A Transsexual Woman on Sexism and the Scapegoating of Femininity, 1st Edition.* Emeryville, CA: Seal Press.

Sewell, A. A. 2017. "Illness Associations of Police Violence: Differential Relationships by Ethnoracial Composition." *Sociological Forum* 32(S1): 975–997.

Sewell, A. A., and Kevin A. Jefferson. 2016. "Collateral Damage: The Health Effects of Invasive Police Encounters in New York City." *Journal of Urban Health* 93(1): 42–67.

Sewell, A. A., Kevin A. Jefferson, and Hedwig Lee. 2016. "Living Under Surveillance: Gender, Psychological Distress, and Stop-Question-and-Frisk Policing in New York City." *Social Science & Medicine* 159: 1–13.

Sewell, Alyasah Ali. 2020. "We Need a 21st Century New Deal." *Contexts*

shuster, stef. 2017. "Punctuating Accountability: How Discursive Aggression Regulates Transgender People." *Gender & Society* 31(4): 481–502.

shuster, stef. 2018. "Passing as Experts in Transgender Medicine." Pp. 74–87 in *The Unfinished Queer Agenda After Marriage*, edited by Angela Jones, Michael W. Yarbrough, and Joseph Nicholas DeFilippis. New York, NY: Routledge.

Simula, Brandy, J. E. Sumerau, and Andrea Miller (eds.). 2019. *Expanding the Rainbow: Exploring the Relationships of Bi+, Polyamorous, Kinky, Ace, Intersex, and Trans People.* Boston, MA: Brill/Sense.

Smolak, Linda and Ruth H. Striegel-Moore. 2001. "Challenging the Myth of the Golden Girl: Ethnicity and Eating Disorders." Pp. 111–132 in *Eating Disorders: Innovative Directions in Research and Practice*, edited by Ruth H. Striegel-Moore and Linda Smolak. Washington, DC: American Psychological Association.

Stryker, Susan. 2008. *Transgender History, 1ˢᵗ edition.* Berkeley, CA: Seal Press.

Sumerau, J. E. 2017. "'I See Monsters': The Role of Rape in my Personal, Professional, and Political Life." In *Negotiating the Emotional Challenges of Conducting Deeply Personal Research*, edited by Alexandra C. H. Nowakowski and J. E. Sumerau. Boca Raton, FL: CRC Press, Taylor and Francis Publishing Group.

Sumerau, J. E. 2018. *Palmetto Rose.* Boston, MA: Brill.

Sumerau, J. E. 2019. "Embodying Nonexistence: Experiencing Cis and Mono Normativities in Everyday Life." Pp. 177–188 in *Body Battlegrounds: Transgressions, Tensions and Trans-formations*, edited by Chris Bobel and Samantha Kwan. Nashville, TN: Vanderbilt University Press.

Sumerau, J. E. 2020. "A Tale of Three Spectrums: Deviating from Normative Treatments of Sex and Gender." *Deviant Behavior* DOI: 10.1080/01639625.2020.1735030.

Sumerau, J. E. and Eric Anthony Grollman. 2018. "Obscuring Oppression: Racism, Cissexism, and the Persistence of Social Inequality." *Sociology of Race and Ethnicity* 4(3): 322–337.

Sumerau, J. E. and Lain A. B. Mathers. 2019. *America Through Transgender Eyes.* Lanham, MD: Rowman & Littlefield.

Sumerau, J. E. and Alexandra C. H. Nowakowski. 2019. "Relational Fluidity: Somewhere Between Polyamory and Monogamy." Pp. 121–132 in *Expanding the Rainbow: Exploring the Relationships of Bi, Pan, Queer, Ace, Intersex, Trans, Poly, and Kinky, Ace, Intersex, and Trans People*, edited by Brandy Simula, Andrea Miller, and J. E. Sumerau. Boston, MA: Brill/Sense.

Sumerau, J. E., Lain A. B. Mathers, and Ryan T. Cragun. 2016. "'I Found God in the Glory Hole': The Moral Career of a Gay Christian." *Sociological Inquiry* 86(4): 618–640.

Sumerau, J. E., Lain A. B. Mathers, Alexandra C. H. Nowakowski, and Ryan T. Cragun. 2017. "Helping Quantitative Sociology Come out of the Closet." *Sexualities* 20(5–6): 644–656.

Sumerau, J. E., Lain A. B. Mathers, and Moon, Dawne. 2019. Foreclosing Fluidity at the Intersection of Gender and Sexual Normativities. *Symbolic Interaction* DOI: 10.1002/symb.43.

Taliaferro, Lindsay A., Brittany M. Harder, Nik M. Lampe, Shannon K. Carter, G. Nic Rider, and Marla E. Eisenberg. 2019. "Social Connectedness Factors that Facilitate Use of Health-care Services: Comparison of Transgender and Gender Nonconforming and Cisgender Adolescents." *The Journal of Pediatrics* 211: 172–178.

Talley, Heather Laine and Monica J. Casper. 2012. "Intersex and Aging: A (Cautionary) Research Agenda." Pp. 270–289 in *Gay, Lesbian, Bisexual & Transgender Aging: Challenges in Research, Practice & Policy*, edited by Tarynn M. Witten and A. Evan Eyler. Baltimore, MD: Johns Hopkins University Press.

Topp, Sarah S. 2019. "Shifting Medical Paradigms: The Evolution of Relationships between Intersex Individuals and Doctors." Pp. 265–277 in *Expanding the Rainbow: Exploring the Relationships of Bi, Pan, Queer, Ace, Intersex, Trans, Poly, and Kink People*, edited by Brandy Simula, Andrea Miller, and J. E. Sumerau. Boston, MA: Brill/Sense.

Ueno, Koji. 2005. "Sexual Orientation and Psychological Distress in Adolescence: Examining Interpersonal Stressors and Social Support Processes." *Social Psychology Quarterly* 68(3): 258–277.

United Nations for LGBT Equality. 2017. "Fact Sheet: Intersex." Retrieved on Feb. 22, 2020 (https://www.unfe.org/wp-content/uploads/2017/05/UNFE-Intersex.pdf).

U.S. Department of Health and Human Services and National Institute on Minority Health and Health Disparities. 2016. "Director's Message: Sexual and Gender Minorities Formally Designated as a Health Disparity Population for Research Purposes." Retrieved on Feb. 22, 2020 (https:// www.nimhd.nih.gov/about/directors-corner/messages/message_10–06–16).

Warner, Michael. 1999. *The Trouble with Normal: Sex, Politics, and the Ethics of Queer Life.* New York, NY: Free Press.

Washington, Harriet A. 2006. *Medical Apartheid: The Dark History of Medical Experimentation on Black Americans from Colonial Times to the Present.* New York, NY: Doubleday

Wenham, Clare, Julia Smith, and Rosemary Morgan. 2020. "COVID-19: The Gendered Impacts of the Outbreak." *The Lancet* 395(10227): 846–848.

West, Candace and Don H. Zimmerman. 1987. "Doing Gender." *Gender & Society* 1(2): 125–51.

Westbrook, Laurel and Aliya Saperstein. 2015. "New Categories Are Not Enough Rethinking the Measurement of Sex and Gender in Social Surveys." *Gender & Society* 29(4): 534–60.

Williams, David R. and Chiquita Collins. 1995. "US Socioeconomic and Racial Differences in Health: Patterns and Explanations." *Annual Review of Sociology* 21(1): 349–386.

Wingo, Erin, Ingraham, Natalie, and Roberts, Sarah C. M. 2018. "Reproductive Healthcare Priorities and Barriers to Effective Care for LGBTQ People Assigned Female at Birth: A Qualitative Study." *Women's Health Issues* 28(4): 350–357.

Yancy, Clyde W. 2020. "COVID-19 and African Americans." *JAMA.* DOI: 10.1001/jama.2020.6548.

Index

About the Authors

Alexandra "Xan" C. H. Nowakowski (they/them) is an assistant professor in geriatrics and behavioral sciences and social medicine at the Florida State University College of Medicine. They are a medical sociologist, public health program evaluator, and community advocate. Their research, teaching, and outreach focus on health equity in aging with chronic disease. They use mixed methods to explore and amplify the experiences of marginalized populations to inform the effective practice of chronic care for people aging with complex health challenges. They hold a PhD and MS in medical sociology from Florida State University, an MPH in health systems and policy from Rutgers University, and a BA in political science from Columbia University. To all of their professional activities, they bring lessons learned from their own lived experience with cystic fibrosis and complex post-traumatic stress disorder. Building on this history, they co-edited *Negotiating the Emotional Challenges of Conducting Deeply Personal Research in Health* with their spouse and frequent collaborator Dr. J. E. Sumerau. They also co-authored the social fiction novel *Other People's Oysters* focused on intergenerational environmental health and aging on Florida's Forgotten Coast. In addition, they co-founded the academic blog Write Where It Hurts focused on scholarship informed by lived experience of trauma, and contribute to a number of other blogs focused on amplifying patient voices in science and medicine. For more information, please visit www.writewhereithurts.net.

J. E. Sumerau (she/her) is an associate professor and the director of applied sociology at the University of Tampa. She is the author of four books and over seventy-five articles and chapters at the intersections of sexualities, gender, health, violence, and religion. She is also the author of five novels focused on LGBTQIA experience in the Southeastern United States. Her latest books include *America through Transgender Eyes* and *Via Chicago*. For more information, please visit www.jsumerau.com or follow her on Twitter @JSumerau.

Nik M. Lampe (they/them) is an award-winning researcher and doctoral candidate in sociology at the University of South Carolina. Their research focuses on the intersections of sex, gender, sexualities, health, and aging in relation to barriers in healthcare access, utilization, and delivery. They have been published in academic journals including *The Journal of Pediatrics*, *Gender & Society*, *The Qualitative Report*, and *Symbolic Interaction*.

www.ingramcontent.com/pod-product-compliance
Lightning Source LLC
Chambersburg PA
CBHW022328280326
41932CB00010B/1264